SAN DIEGO

PROPERTY OF
NATIONAL UNIVERSITY
LIBRARY

Trauma, Trance, and Transformation: A Clinical Guide to Hypnotherapy

Trauma, Trance, and Transformation

A Clinical Guide to Hypnotherapy

✦✦

M. Gerald Edelstien, M.D.

BRUNNER/MAZEL, *Publishers* • New York

Library of Congress Cataloging in Publication Data

Edelstien, M. Gerald, 1928-
  Trauma, trance, and transformation.

  Bibliography: p.
  Includes index.
  1. Hypnotism—Therapeutic use.   I. Title.
[DNLM: 1. Hypnosis. WM 415 E21t]
RC495.E33   615.8'512   81-10175
ISBN 0-87630-278-9   AACR2

Copyright © 1981 by M. GERALD EDELSTIEN

Published by
BRUNNER/MAZEL, INC.
19 Union Square
New York, New York 10003

All rights reserved. No part of this book may be reproduced
by any process whatsoever, without the written permission of
the publisher.

MANUFACTURED IN THE UNITED STATES OF AMERICA

I wish to express my sincere appreciation to that large number of talented men and women who attempted to teach me many things about this world in which we live.

I also wish to thank George and Ira Gershwin for their song, "It Ain't Necessarily So."

FOREWORD

Trauma, Trance, and Transformation arrives on the therapeutic scene at a time when interest in the clinical values and applications of hypnosis is at a new level of intensity.

If hypnosis is to qualify as an effective form of helping, it must demonstrate its ability to do a job more quickly, more thoroughly, and more lastingly than other forms of therapy. Potentially, hypnosis can accomplish these aims, provided it is adapted to the needs of the patient by a skilled, experienced operator within the context of an integrated treatment plan.

Because hypnosis is capable of promoting relaxation, of rendering the individual more susceptible to suggestion, and of facilitating closer contact with the inner self, advantage may be taken of these characteristics in the management of certain emotional problems. Symptomatic disturbances produced or aggravated by anxiety and tension may be relieved, and destructive habit patterns reorganized through hypnorelaxation and hypnosuggestion. Where therapy is short-term and directed toward abbreviated objectives, hypnosis, utilized properly, can expedite treatment by encouraging rapport, stimulating emotional catharsis, catalyzing the placebo effect and hastening other non-specific therapeutic elements. In longer-term reconstructive therapy, the periodic induction of hypnosis may be helpful toward dissipating resistance and obstructions to communication, augmenting dreaming, accelerating the remembering of important developmental incidents, activating transference, and helping working-through. When a patient seems to have reached a stalemate in therapy, hypnosis may open up new dimensions for exploration and understanding. It may propagate the translation of insight into action.

Despite its recognized usefulness, controversy exists, even among the experts, about many aspects of hypnosis, such as its indications and contraindications; the most effective methods for inducing a trance; the utility of testing for trance depth; whether non-susceptible persons can be trained to become good subjects; whether trance depth is a fixed or fluctuating characteristic; the relationship of trance depth to therapeutic effectiveness; dangers inherent in the use of hypnosis; utility and permanence of hypnotic symptom removal; hypnotic powers to persuade subjects to commit anti-social acts; the nature of hypnotically induced amnesia; the likelihood of encouraging dependency through hypnotherapy; whether responses to hypnosis give clues to diagnosis and selection of preferred therapeutic interventions; how hypnosis may be employed most propitiously to facilitate therapeutic interventions; and the utility of such hypnoanalytic techniques as dream induction, fantasy stimulation, guided imagery, automatic writing, regression and revivification, and the induction of experimental conflicts.

The virtue of the present volume is that it addresses itself to many of these questions. It additionally provides an excellent vista of the leading uncovering, attenuating, and relearning techniques in an unpretentious and practical way. The revival of interest in hypnosis is not a fortuitous happening; it signals accumulating evidence of the value of hypnosis in medicine and psychiatry.

Since World War II hypnosis has experienced a steady rise in favor. This has been the product of dedicated workers in the field who, through their writings and teachings, have helped hypnosis find its rightful place in the family of serviceable methodologies.

Perhaps the most diligent of workers was Milton Erickson, who contributed a vast body of techniques and research findings and who, more than any other person in modern times, has stimulated continuing interest in a field traditionally enveloped in superstition and magic. His methods, uniquely his own, acted as a conduit for his forceful and persuasive personality. These have been studied and analyzed by Haley, Rossi, Bandler and Grinder with the object of distilling out principles suitable for the therapeutic armamentaria of the mental health professions. Not all therapists will acquire the sensitivity and perceptiveness that characterized Erickson's ability to harmonize his techniques with the shifting defensive maneuvers of his patients, and in this way circumvent or resolve their resistance. However, with practice, therapists may be able to coordinate with their own unique styles of operation the interventions of Erickson and other authorities in the field, including those methods described so clearly by the author of this book.

Most of the work done with hypnosis is relatively uncomplicated, being bracketed to symptom-oriented and problem-solving methodologies. Greater problems will be encountered where hypnosis is employed with psychoanalytic techniques in methods labeled "hypnoanalysis." The literature is replete with many cleverly devised stratagems devised to explore in hypnosis undercurrent moods, attitudes, impulses, and conflicts. A good number of these schemes, such as those utilizing regression and revivification, complex post-hypnotic suggestions, and the setting up of experimental conflicts, require a deep or somnambulistic trance and hence are limited to a small percentage of patients. Of greater utility are hypnoanalytic interventions that can be employed in light or medium hypnosis. Among these are "ideomotor signaling," "the affect bridge" and "ego state therapy," all of which are explicated in the volume. Here the "unconscious" and the various personality configurations ("ego states") within the individual are invited to speak out as independent entities. There is some resemblance to methods utilized during gestalt therapy, transactional analysis, and psychodrama. Some of the techniques are highly theatrical and undoubtedly appeal to the histrionic pretensions of certain patients who will enthusiastically enter into play-acting and role-playing. One should not deceive oneself regarding the authenticity of the material emerging in the trance—the fascinating narratives of previous lives, the confidences of intrauterine existence, the upheaval of the birth experience, and the tortured portrayal of growing up that are so thrillingly and convincingly recounted by some patients. This content should never be taken at face value but rather dealt with as symbolic offerings, very much like fantasies or dreams. Through proper interpretation, interesting insights may emerge that may be helpful in the working-through process. But even where the exposed content is an accurate reflection of previous development experiences or of verifiable unconscious conflicts, the disclosures will not necessarily have a positive therapeutic effect. On the contrary, they may stimulate resistance and even intensify the very symptoms for which the patient seeks help. This is not necessarily bad, for in the overcoming of resistance we have an opportunity of scoring reconstructive gains. What becomes apparent with experience is that a thorough grounding in dynamic theory and practice is most advantageous where a therapist has any aspirations of working hypnoanalytically with patients.

A final caveat may be in order. The most serious threat to the acceptance of hypnosis by the mental health professions is not from its critics who equate it with brainwashing, but from its overenthusiastic supporters who claim for it miraculous powers. Hypnosis is no miracle monger. Indiscriminate use will relegate it to the trash heap of outmoded and antiquated therapies which seems to have been its historical destiny. But employed conservatively as an adjunct, it can play an important part in shortening all forms of psychotherapy and making them more serviceable and effective.

Considering all these circumstances—the very real therapeutic benefits along with the dangers of misuse and overestimation—it is fortunate, indeed, that this volume is available as a stimulating, clearly presented, and exceedingly useful guide to the effective application of hypnosis in therapy. Dr. Edelstien has made a very real contribution to this important field.

LEWIS R. WOLBERG, M.D.
Chairman, Postgraduate Center
for Mental Health (New York)

CONTENTS

    The Case of Helen 125

7. PUTTING IT ALL TOGETHER 127
    Selection of Patients 130
    Cases Not Requiring Uncovering Techniques 131
    Removal of Bad Habits 132
    Engendering Good Habits 133
    Reducing Affect from Known Sources 134
    Relieving Insomnia 135
    Selection of Uncovering Techniques 135
    Selection of Affect Attenuation Techniques 136
    Selection of Relearning Techniques 137
    Termination 138

8. CONCLUSION 141

    Bibliography 145

    Index 147

INTRODUCTION

❖❖

This volume has been written in the belief it can demonstrate that hypnotic techniques, used in a systematic manner, will greatly enrich the armamentarium of those therapists who have recognized the value of brief psychotherapy. The techniques are easily learned, are highly effective in a broad spectrum of clinical disorders, and can be utilized by almost any psychotherapist, whatever his theoretical background might be.

It is written in the hope that it will aid those already using hypnosis and can persuade some who are not; however, in regard to the latter group, it has been my observation that each of us tends to believe the system we already practice is superior to all other systems of therapy.

It is natural that we should believe this. for there is little reason for any of us to practice one way if we believe another way to be better. It's likely, however, that serious consideration is rarely given to the possibility that another way might be better. We are taught, we practice in accordance with our teachings, we obtain reasonably good results, and those good results convince us of the veracity of our teachings.

We also have failures when we practice according to our teachings. We interpret our failures as the improper application of what we were taught or, more malignantly, as the patient's inability to utilize therapy. We hear of an innovator's good results and pass them off as superficial improvements not worthy of serious consideration. We hear of his failures and offer them as proof of the fallacy of his system. Ralph Greenson (1967) alluded to this when he wrote, "The secluded innovators are prone to become 'wild analysts,' while the conservatives, due to their own insularity, tend to become rigid with orthodoxy" (p. 2).

But how can the therapist who has not yet become rigid with orthodoxy determine if another way is better? Research on the relative efficacy of differing forms of therapy has yielded no compelling statistics. The behavioral therapists, perhaps more than others, have offered statistics, but their statistics have not compelled colleagues to discontinue insight-oriented therapy in favor of progressive desensitization in the treatment of phobias. Despite what many consider to be the demonstrated efficacy of tricyclics in the management of depression, many others do not use them, believing analysis of underlying dynamics is the only acceptable treatment for this malady.

Despite the questionable validity of personal anecdotes, we apparently tend to rely upon those more than upon statistics concerning the "talking therapies." When faced with such statistics, we find fault with the statistical methods used or disagree with the criteria for cure. We reject the conclusions and continue basing our practices on personal anecdotes. We also rely upon the influence of respected teachers, even, perhaps, when their teachings occasionally are contrary to our own clinical observations. We rationalize these discrepancies by assuming we have done something wrong, rather than face the possibility that the teachings were faulty.

Increasingly, however, concerns are being raised about the doctrines we were taught. Theory is being questioned and traditional techniques are being attacked. For example, David H. Malan (1980), one of the major proponents of briefer therapy, has written:

> It needs to be stated categorically that in the early part of this century Freud unwittingly took a wrong turning which led to disastrous consequences for the future of psychotherapy. This was to react to increasing resistance with increased passivity—eventually adopting the technique of free association on the part of the patient, and the role of "passive sounding board," free floating attention, and infinite patience on the part of the therapist.
> The consequences have been strenuously ignored or denied by generations of analysts and dynamic psychotherapists, but are there for all to see. The most obvious effect has been an enormous increase in the duration of treatment—from a few weeks or months to many years. A less obvious development is that the method has become, to say the least, of doubtful therapeutic effectiveness.

Dissatisfaction with traditional therapy, a dissatisfaction affecting therapists and patients alike, has given rise to many new modes of therapy. Presumably the practitioners of each mode cherish it, while the practitioners of other modes find it lacking, if not contemptible. It is true, I believe, that we tend to overvalue our own and undervalue the others'.

Many of the newer modes disappear in time; others prosper and prove their worth. In regarding them, it might serve us well to heed a quote from Freud, written in his introduction to Bernheim's book on therapeutic hypnosis. In it he is pleading with those who reject hypnosis out of ignorance: "It remains true in scientific matters it is always experience, and never authority without experience, that gives the final verdict, whether in favor or against."

It is my plan to present another modality for brief therapy. I cannot speak from authority, but I can speak from experience, and to me the verdict is clear: Profound and lasting changes can be effected by a systematic use of hypnotic techniques which enable the therapist to achieve the same results that are derived from more conventional therapies. The results may be obtained more easily and more rapidly, and that is satisfying to the patient and therapist alike.

CHAPTER ONE

Historical Notes

✠✠✠

The history of hypnosis in the practice of medicine is long, and although it is also interesting, it is not my purpose to dwell at length on the past. There are, however, certain highlights worth repeating, for they demonstrate the tenacity, perhaps even the irrationality, with which our profession tends to cling to established practices rather than give due credit to innovators.

Franz Anton Mesmer (1734-1815) is regarded by many as the father of modern medical hypnosis. He is also regarded by many as a charlatan, and that alleged sin of the father has brought unwarranted discredit to generations of hypnotherapists who succeeded him. Vincent Buranelli's carefully researched biography of Mesmer, *The Wizard from Vienna* (1975), indicates that he was no charlatan. He treated all who came to him, rich and poor alike; he made no secret of what he believed or practiced; he steadfastly denied mystic powers; he repeatedly offered to present his theory and performance to the scientific community for its consideration. His two greatest sins were a waspish personality and a belief in an unsound theory, vices not unknown in his day, nor in ours.

After graduating from the University of Vienna, one of the finest medical schools in the world at that time, Mesmer published his doctoral thesis, *The Influence of the Planets on the Human Body*. Medical science being what it was in that day, his was considered a rational thesis. After several years of a traditional and respectable practice, Mesmer began experimenting with magnets to treat cases of hysteria and obtained some remarkable cures.

He evolved a theory of a universal fluid which ebbed and flowed throughout the body, causing or relieving symptoms, and believed magnetic influences could alter the course of that fluid. He soon discovered mineral magnets were unnecessary to produce the cures and came to believe certain persons, himself included, possessed an animal magnetism which permitted them to cure "nervous" disorders.

His many successes, frequently with patients who had not responded to the medical ministrations of more conventional physicians, soon brought him so many patients he was unable to treat them all on an individual basis. He invented the baquet, a bathtub-like apparatus with metal rods and iron filings attached, and had patients sit around the tub, applying the rods to the affected parts of their bodies. Thus, he was not only the father of medical hypnosis, but also, in his own crude way, the father of group therapy.

As his patients sat around the tub, he would stroll past in silken robes, pointing his magnetic wand at them. Many would go into a crisis, which ranged from a simple exacerbation of their symptoms to severe convulsions. After the crisis, improvement began.

Although he was eminently successful in his practice, his bitter disappointment at not gaining recognition from his colleagues led him to leave Vienna for Paris, where he again gained an enormous following of patients and again reaped disdain from his fellow physicians. A scientific commission was appointed to investigate his claims and the commission, which included Benjamin Franklin and Dr. Guillotine as its members, declared he indeed effected remarkable cures, but merely as a result of suggestion.

Mesmer left Paris in disgrace. His colleagues, who practiced the acceptable arts of bleeding and blistering, ignored his cures and rejected his technique because it was "only suggestion."

Some seventy years later, in 1846, James Esdaile, a Scottish surgeon practicing in India, published *Mesmerism in India,* a book in which he described several thousand minor operations and approximately three hundred major ones, all done painlessly with the patient mesmerized. Despite the fact that chemical anesthesia was not yet in popular usage and despite the fact that other surgeons still performed operations while their patients endured horrible pain, Esdaile was ridiculed because what he was doing was "only mesmerism."

Almost another seventy years later, during World War I, and again during World War II, the thousands of psychiatric casualties far outweighed the traditional psychiatric treatment time available. It was found that hypnosis could often relieve the battlefield neuroses in only one or a few sessions. Today, however, few colleagues use this modality to treat traumatic neuroses. Perhaps this is because they believe traumatic neuroses in civilians are different from traumatic neuroses in military men, but more likely this proven method of treatment is rejected because it is "only hypnosis."

These three historical items support the adage that those who do not learn from history are bound to repeat it. For any serious psychotherapist, however, there is one more historical event deserving further scrutiny: Freud's rejection of hypnosis.

In *Analysis Terminable and Interminable,* Freud (1937) wrote, "Someday the pure gold of psychoanalysis may have to be alloyed with the copper of suggestion." My analytic friends consider this a great compliment to psychoanalysis; the iconoclast might wonder if it really is. After all, pure gold is uncommonly heavy, inordinately expensive, and far too soft to be of much practical value until it is alloyed with some baser metal. Without dwelling further on that quotation, let us briefly examine Freud's use of hypnosis.

By today's standards Freud would be considered a poor hypnotist. In 1891 he had written, "The technique of hypnotizing is just as difficult a medical procedure as any other" (p. 105), and in his *Five Lectures* (1910) he stated, "But I soon came to dislike hypnosis.... When I found that, in spite of all my efforts, I could not succeed in bringing more than a fraction of my patients into a hypnotic state, I determined to give up hypnosis."

It is hard to imagine why Freud had such difficulties. He had studied under both Charcot and Bernheim and had even written the introduction to the German edition of Bernheim's book. In that book, originally published in 1884, Bernheim had described several simple inductions, one of which consisted of nothing more than "Look at me and think of nothing but sleep. Your eyelids begin to feel heavy, your eyes tired. They begin to wink, they are getting moist, you cannot see distinctly. They are closed." Bernheim (1884) quoted statistics from Liébault (1880), who found only 27 refractory cases in 1,012 subjects.

Whatever the reasons for Freud's difficulty in inducing the hypnotic state, he was further restricted by the therapeutic techniques then available. His only tools were direct suggestion and abreaction, techniques which are still employed today, but both are of limited usefulness, and unless complemented by more modern techniques, will generally produce only modest successes. To compare Freud's methods of hypnotherapy to modern methods would be somewhat akin to comparing his usage of psychopharmacology to that which is available today.

I do not know if the induction techniques used today are truly an improvement on those used by Bernheim almost one hundred years ago, but instead of their being as difficult as any other medical procedure, as Freud described them, modern techniques can easily produce a usable trance state within five minutes with 90 to 95 percent of subjects. Some induction techniques can do the same within a matter of seconds. The therapeutic techniques have improved enormously since Freud and any psychotherapist who still rejects the use of hypnosis on the basis of Freud's discontent is operating with outmoded data.

Even though Freud was severely restricted in methods of induction and in methods of utilizing the hypnotic state, there may well have been more compelling reasons for his abandonment of this modality. In his autobiography, Freud wrote that while he was using hypnosis to treat a female patient for pain, she suddenly awoke and threw her arms around him. The coincidental appearance of a house servant "fortunately" saved him from a painful discussion of that event, and from that time on, there was a "tacit understanding" that hypnotic therapy would be discontinued. He believed he now understood the "mysterious element" behind hypnosis, and "In order to exclude it, or at all events to isolate it, it was necessary to abandon hypnosis."

Hypnosis and Freud both apparently suffered from this incident, but psychoanalysis advanced significantly, for this led to Freud's understanding of transference. His stated reasons for abandoning hypnosis, however, may not have been completely accurate, but may have been, at least in part, pure rationalization. Jerome Schneck (1954) in "Countertransference in Freud's Rejection of Hypnosis" suggests another possible motive. That motive is easily surmised from the title of his article and is related directly to Freud's reaction upon finding himself suddenly and embarrassingly embraced.

Whatever reasons Freud had, I believe his abandonment of hypnosis has had much to do with the fact that orthodox therapists now regard hypnosis with disdain. Modern therapists can reject or modify others of Freud's beliefs in the light of more recent findings, but most have difficulty in reappraising his assessment of hypnosis. In some instances this may be because they are unaware of the advances made; in some, because of rationalizations of their own; and in some, because of an honest admission that they are afraid to try it. Few know enough about the subject to reach a thoughtful opinion.

Freud is no irrefutable source on all matters pertaining to analysis. Certainly he is no irrefutable source on the subject of hypnosis. It is entirely conceivable there are no irrefutable sources in our field and, unscientific though it may be, perhaps we are stuck with relying upon personal anecdotes to large measure. If that is true, then it may also be true that the anecdotes upon which we rely need not come only from the most prestigious of sources, nor must they be shrouded in the most convoluted of theories. Simple techniques of therapy which work well, albeit without a profound theoretical basis, should be given as much serious consideration as complicated techniques endowed with their own complicated theories. Perhaps it is not irrational to use final therapeutic results as the measure of a system's worth. Mesmer and Esdaile would not have been disgraced for their efforts and countless patients would have been saved incalculable suffering.

CHAPTER TWO

Theoretical Notes

✤✤

Generally one expects a book on hypnosis to offer a definition of the phenomenon and a theory as to how it works. This book will offer neither. Although there is no shortage of definitions nor any shortage of theories, none is truly satisfactory, so they will not be included. There are those who claim there is no such thing as a hypnotic state and no one can prove them wrong. Still, the concept of there being such a state is a useful concept; patients respond as though the state does exist and, consequently, good therapy can be done. That to some, most certainly to the patient, is more important than a theory or a definition.

By the same token, we should realize that no one can prove the existence of an id or a superego. Certainly there are no x-ray demonstrations of either, and not once has one been recovered at autopsy. Still, the concept of there being an id and a superego is useful; patients respond as though such entities exist and, consequently, good therapy can be done.

It is highly important to recognize, when considering the use of hypnosis in psychotherapy, that hypnosis per se is not a treatment; it is a series of techniques. There are already a number of techniques used in a more traditional style. There is free association. There are interpretations of dreams, fantasies, and slips of the tongue. There are analyses of resistances and of transferences and, of course, there is the working-through process.

These techniques are honored not only because of their longevity, but also because they work, sometimes. The techniques to be described in the following chapters also work, sometimes. But there are important and exciting differences in the ways in which they work—comfort, speed, and efficiency being not the least important of those differences.

Before looking at the techniques, though, let us consider what therapy does, or at least what occurs in the patient that enables change to take place. Most therapists tend to squirm uncomfortably if asked directly what they believe happens within the patient during successful therapy. Before reading any further, perhaps it would be interesting to define the process yourself if you have not done so previously. Of course, in order to define what happens in therapy, it is first necessary to define what sort of therapy—insight-oriented, supportive, behavior modification? Try each, or others.

Very simply stated, I believe there are basically four events occurring in an insight-oriented therapy, and one or more of those events occurring in most of the other therapies. The four are: 1) uncovering of repressed material; 2) some reexperiencing of the affect associated to that material; 3) attenuation of that affect; and 4) learning how to meet new situations unencumbered by the repressed material or its attendant affect.

In their "Preliminary Communication," Breuer and Freud (1893) maintained:

> Each individual hysterical symptom immediately and promptly disappeared when we had succeeded in bringing clearly to light

the memory of the event by which it was provoked (uncovering) and in arousing the accompanying affect (reexperiencing), and when the patient had described that event in the greatest possible detail and had put the affect into words (attenuation).

As we know, Freud later abandoned hypnosis and, from 1912 on, the consistent analysis of transference and resistance became the central element of the psychoanalytic process. It is important to realize, however, that analysis of a resistance is primarily a technique designed to facilitate the recovery of repressed material (uncovering) and/or its attendant affect (reexperiencing). Analysis of a transference is only more of the same, done from a somewhat different perspective. Greenson (1967, p. 189) states, more elegantly, "It is recognized the transference neurosis offers the patient the most important instrumentality for gaining access to the warded off past pathogenic experience." As the material that had been repressed and the affect which had been defended against surface again and again during the analysis, attenuation occurs, and the working-through process permits relearning.

In supportive therapy, during which the therapist acts primarily as an auxiliary ego for the patient, most of what happens is relearning. Here the patient learns to face new situations differently because the therapist teaches him, and he is relatively unencumbered by the old conflicts because he is following the dictates of his guru. In confrontation therapies, the main emphasis appears to be getting the patient to admit to and abreact an affect, most frequently anger. Thus, reexperiencing and attenuation are the primary ingredients of this therapy. Perhaps it is less effective than one would hope because the anger abreacted was not the primary affect, but was secondary to the grief, fear, shame, etc., which was provoked by some important figure or situation.

I have not attempted to look at all the different behavior modification techniques from this viewpoint, but with progressive desensitization, in which the patient is exposed to gradual increments of a noxious affect, we see attenuation and relearning. The behaviorists say once behavior has changed, there is frequently insight into the origin of the symptom (uncovering). Perhaps little reexperiencing occurs for attenuation has already been accomplished and there may not be much of the original affect remaining.

Judd Marmor (1980) lists what he considers to be the important elements in the psychotherapeutic process:

1) "Release of emotional tension in the context of hope and expectation of receiving help." I would assume this means both the release of tension that inhibits the recovery of re-pressed material (uncovering) and the release of tension that follows the recovery of the repressed material (reex-periencing and attenuation).
2) "Cognitive learning about the basis for the patient's diffi-culties" (uncovering).
3) "Operant reconditioning toward more adaptive patterns of behavior by means of explicit or implicit approval-disap-proval cues, and also through corrective emotional experi-ences in therapy" (relearning and attenuation).
4) "Suggestion and persuasion, overt or covert." I would con-sider this part of the therapist's technique, not something that happens within the patient.
5) "Identification with the therapist or other group members." (Attenuation—i.e., if the therapist doesn't feel some act or impulse was so terrible, the patient, identifying with him, will begin to feel it wasn't all that bad; relearning—i.e., if the therapist can perform in some given way, so can the patient.)
6) "Repeated reality testing or rehearsal of the new adaptive techniques" (relearning).

If recovery of repressed material, reliving of the affect connected to that material, attenuation of the affect, and relearning how to cope with new situations are indeed the essence of what occurs in an insight-oriented therapy, and if it can be shown that currently available hypnotic techniques can accomplish those four steps more effectively than traditional techniques, then one of the major ob-jections the traditionalist has toward hypnosis logically should be removed. Another objection will quickly arise, however, for it will soon be found that the repressed material uncovered by these techniques may differ from what the traditionalist would have expected. This will become readily apparent as I present case histories and may cause the traditionalist to claim the material recovered is not truly the source of the neurosis but is merely a screen to camouflage the true source.

But if the patient presents unexpected data as the source of his difficulties, what is to be done with those data? There are at least two possibilities: The material can be discredited because it does not fit the accepted theories, or the theories can be discredited because they are not consonant with the data. The more traditional the therapist, the more inclined he is to discredit the data. He will explain, "This is nothing more than a screen memory," or "This more superficial (partial, inaccurate) interpretation only prevents the patient from reexperiencing the true conflicts. Any apparent improvement is due to bolstering his defenses." This therapist will find much support from his colleagues.

The less traditional the therapist, the easier it is for him to reject the theory, but then he is in the uncomfortable position of doing work for which there is, as yet, no sound theoretical basis. That is not altogether an untenable spot, for there is precedent for theory evolving from clinical observation. Further observation may alter or even refute whatever theory is evolved. Here it is important for us to remember that a theory is not necessarily the same as a fact. Webster includes among his definitions of theory "a speculative plan, conjecture, a guess." We have seen psychoanalytic theories about the origin of mania and of (some) depressions become less tenable as observations of genetics and of neurotransmitters become more refined. Freud himself refined his own theories as he accumulated more data. It seems reasonable, therefore, to be open to the possibility that other theories may need revision as more data accumulate in the field of behavioral sciences.

To the traditionalist who insists he always finds what traditional theory states he will find, I offer no disagreement. I am fairly certain a therapist can almost always "uncover" whatever he expects to be there. In coming to this conclusion, I thought of three therapists I knew, one of whom almost always found narcissistic problems in his patients, one of whom almost always found dependency problems, and one of whom almost always found repressed anger. I postulated that each of them could find, in the same patient, whichever one of those three dynamics he was most interested in finding.

Having no access to actually hearing those therapists in operation, but having ready access to my own imagination, it was easy to conceive of how this might be managed. Were the patient to make the simple statement, "I was upset when my mother left me with the baby-sitter," each therapist, perhaps unaware of what he was doing, could easily lead the patient into one of three different directions. The narcissistic therapist could say, "You were upset when your mother left *you*?" The dependency therapist could say, "You were upset when your *mother* left you?" The angry therapist could say, "You were *upset* when your mother left you?" The inflection need be only slight to have the suggestive effect that further discussion should proceed along (the therapist's) predetermined lines. A written transcript would not display this coaxing to the "right" information.

Even the therapist who merely says, "Hmm," to the patient's productions can easily lead the patient in predetermined directions. If the flow heads in the "right" direction, the therapist's "hmm" will sound like, "Hmm, that's interesting, tell me more." If the direction appears "wrong," the "hmm" will sound like, "Hmm, that's boring, talk about something else."

The traditionalist can easily raise the objections: My ideas of how a therapist can lead the patient to the "right" data are mere speculation, and only an unskilled therapist would do such a thing, even if it were possible. To the first objection I can only say, "Hmm." To the second objection I would like to quote Sigmund Freud. In "The Analysis of a Phobia in a Five-Year-Old Boy" (1909), the case which "established" the dynamics of a phobia, he wrote, "It is true that during the analysis Hans had to be told many things which he could not say himself, that he had to be presented with his thoughts which he had so far shown no signs of possessing and that his attention had to be turned in the direction from which his father was expecting something to come."

Wolpe and Rachman have written a thought-provoking article, "Psychoanalytic Evidence: A Critique Based on Freud's Case of Little Hans" (1960), in which they look carefully and critically at the evidence used to prove the theory. The fact that Hans was actually frightened by a falling horse just prior to his developing a phobia toward horses was ignored in favor of material for which the therapist was looking. His father indoctrinated Hans as to what certain symbols meant (to the father), and later, when Hans repeated those meanings, it was taken as evidence of Hans' unconscious processes. Hans' spontaneous comments contradicting some of the theoretical beliefs were ignored. Hans was asked many leading questions, some of them repeatedly. His later agreements were considered confirmations, while his disagreements were defined as resistances. Using those rules of evidence, it would be possible for anyone to prove any theory he chose. Those who don't believe are merely being resistant.

To demonstrate the above points from a more modern perspective, let's take a brief look at *The Psychoanalytic Process: A Case Illustration.* This remarkably honest book, in which Paul Dewald (1972) presents transcripts from his analysis of a young lady, has many examples. Session 145 (p. 211) begins:

> P: When I lie down here I picture my house in Evanston and I feel as if I'm right there. (Elaborates.)—I feel as if I'm a baby in a crib and yet I'm trying to live like I'm twenty-seven. I feel like someone has a stick in my throat and my stomach is gnawing as if I hadn't eaten. It's all so real! And yet I just ate breakfast a little while ago. I feel huge. I get bigger with every bite of food that I take.—Now I'm back to reliving the time when I was a baby. What's the advantage of all of this? It's really hell!—I feel such hostility! I get so mad! I feel as if I could go crazy! (Elaborates.) Now I have an urge to scream and yell right here on the floor.—I have a terrible feeling in my stomach and it's all sour and hot and it gnaws at me. I feel sick and I can't talk.

A: What are your associations to this sick feeling?

Why did the therapist choose to make this particular intervention and fail to make others when the patient paused or changed topics? He doesn't explain, although most certainly it is not from lack of candor, for elsewhere he clearly describes his reasoning, even when he considers his interventions to have been ill-advised. My purpose in offering this illustration is not to fault Dewald, but to point out there were many opportunities to make other appropriate interventions, each of which would presumably have led the patient in another direction. Both the angry therapist and the dependent therapist would have had the chance to seek elaboration on the anger or the dependency. Other therapists would have pursued her feeling that she could go crazy. Still others would have questioned her inability to talk at that point. I contend that free associations are less free than we might imagine and the therapist definitely directs them toward his anticipated goal.

Dewald himself clearly recognizes this possibility, for he writes, with charitable regard for the competency of his fellow therapists (p. 621):

> By virtue of his clinical experience, theoretical knowledge, and emotional neutrality, the analyst can frequently recognize derivatives of specific unconscious conflicts long before the patient develops such recognition. By emphasizing these elements unduly he might thus through indirect suggestion to a significant extent focus the patient's interest and attention in the directions which he sees as most significant in terms of his theoretical understanding. Although his clinical and theoretical understanding will cause the analyst to exercise selectivity in his interactions with the patient, he must be aware of the potency of this form of indirect suggestion. Otherwise he may find himself in the situation of unconsciously suggesting material to the patient, and then, hearing it repeated back to him, mistake this for a spontaneous confirmation of his ideas.

Had the father of Little Hans had access to this warning, would the current analytic theory of phobias still be the same? Another warning, perhaps, could also have been added. Dewald states, ". . . the analyst can frequently recognize derivatives of specific unconscious conflicts. . . ." The analyst could be warned that what he *assumes* to be derivatives may in reality be remnants of a conflict long since resolved, or even his own association to the patient's words, based on his own theoretical constructs, if not on his own unresolved conflicts.

CHAPTER THREE

✦✦✦

The Trance

✦✦✦

✿✿

There are a number of misconceptions surrounding hypnosis which cause a small percentage of patients and a high percentage of therapists to be wary of using it. Generally, simple, brief explanations are sufficient to reassure the patients; therapists require more reassurance. This is understandable; there is more motivation for giving up unwanted symptoms than for giving up long-cherished beliefs. Additionally, the patients' misconceptions have come primarily from nothing more sacred than poor movies and bad television programs, while the therapists' misconceptions have come from respected teachers.

Naturally, therapists are concerned about the contraindications they were taught about hypnosis, but, despite what they were taught, basically there are only three: the therapist who doesn't know how to use it, the patient who doesn't want to use it, and the patient who wants to use it for unethical or unrealistic purposes. The first contraindication is always relative, the second is often temporary, and the third is easily recognized.

Regarding the therapist who doesn't know how to use hypnosis, there are two different areas of knowledge required: hypnotic techniques per se and the area of expertise in which it is to be used. Specifically, it would be unwise for anyone to use hypnosis for psychotherapy unless he already knows basic principles of psychotherapy.

In respect to the patient's unwillingness to use hypnosis, there are those whose religious beliefs preclude the use of it. It is questionable whether one should attempt to alter those beliefs; personally, I would not, although I have seen patients who believed their religion forbade it, but upon asking their ministers learned it was acceptable for medical purposes. Those who are unwilling because of their misconceptions about hypnosis can be relieved of those misconceptions. Those who are unwilling because they fear some terrible secret will emerge can be reassured with total honesty that such an occurrence is extremely rare. There are many who are reluctant to try because they fear they will fail to respond adequately. To relieve their performance anxiety, these patients are told it may not work, and if it doesn't, more conventional methods can be used, but the odds greatly favor its working and there's little to lose except the few minutes it takes to find out.

As for patients who seek hypnosis for unethical or unrealistic purposes, a few case examples will illustrate how easily recognizable those are: There have been patients who wished to develop extraordinary physical strengths or skills, or photographic memories. There was a paranoid patient who wished me to hypnotize his wife in his presence so he could learn if she had been unfaithful to him. There was a schizophrenic patient who wanted me to teach him self-hypnosis so he could levitate himself. (He rose from his chair when I refused.)

The contraindications to hypnosis that were taught during my psychiatric residency proved to be gross exaggerations. Schizophrenic patients do not lose all sense of ego boundaries and disintegrate into florid psychoses. Patients who are latently homosexual or actively homosexual do not go into homosexual panics. Hysterics do not believe they've been seduced, for although it does feel good to be hypnotized, it doesn't feel that good, even to a hysteric. Dependent patients do not become more dependent. I say that patients do not do these things, but that, of course, depends upon the therapist's doing his job properly. All of those undesirable outcomes could occur with hypnosis, just as they can and do with more traditional therapies.

Psychotherapists who are unfamiliar with hypnosis still labor under the belief that nothing is accomplished but temporary symptom removal. They believe the underlying dynamics which gave birth to those symptoms are untouched, and consequently either the original symptom will return or an even more horrendous one will take its place. Freud probably deserves much credit for perpetuating this belief, for much of his work with hypnosis did involve simply attempting to suggest the symptoms away, and indeed they often returned. It should be remembered, however, that there are better techniques available today than Freud had at his disposal. It should also be remembered that the return of symptoms is not unknown with traditional therapy, either after termination or just prior to termination, as a resistance to the termination; the latter is uncommon with hypnotherapy. In traditional therapy, symptoms also appear again and again during the working-through phase. This can be true with hypnosis, but the working-through process can be accomplished more quickly with hypnosis than without it.

Patients, unencumbered by theoretical concerns, are apt to worry about more "practical" considerations. Will they be certain to come out of the trance? Will they do or say things they will later regret? Will they know what is happening and will they be able to remember it later? Will hypnosis make them weak-willed?

Patients do come out of the trance. On rare occasions they may resist, but this should be no cause for alarm since it can be dealt with easily. First, the patient should be asked why he is not awakening; if he gives a reason, his reason is given proper attention. For

example, a young man did not come out of the trance when I suggested he do so. I asked why not, and he replied, "When I was hypnotized by Dr. . . . ., I was told when it was time to come out I
would let my right arm rise above my head, and then I would
awaken." I instructed him to let his right arm rise above his head
and awaken; he promptly did both.

The only other patient who gave me similar trouble in twenty-
three years of experience would always take fifteen minutes or more
to awaken after I instructed her to do so. She would never give a
reason for the delay. Finally, I told her, "Look, your taking this
long to awaken each time throws me behind schedule, so if you
don't come out of it right now, I won't use hypnosis with you anymore." There were no problems after that. William Bryant taught
a more commercial variation of the same process: "Okay, you can
stay in it as long as you want, but you're using my office, so I'll have
to charge you . . . . dollars an hour." He said his patients would
awaken within two or three minutes.

The question of whether a subject will do things that are nor-
mally against his will is debatable. Some authorities in the field believe a subject can be made to do such things; many authorities
disagree. There have been experiments in which volunteer subjects
while hypnotized simulated antisocial acts or attempted to pick up
dangerous snakes shielded by "invisible" glass, but that is not the
same as having a subject commit an actual crime or truly injure
himself in response to a suggestion. If any hypnotists have led subjects to criminal behavior or to self-injury, they have taken care not
to report it in the journals.

It is likely, however, that some subjects may do things under
hypnosis they would not do under more ordinary circumstances.
Once hypnotized, it is easier to disclaim responsibility for their own
actions and claim, "He made me do it." Those poor "innocents"
who walk onto the stage with a nightclub hypnotist illustrate this
point well. They display the exhibitionist behavior the hypnotist
suggests, willingly accept his suggestions for amnesia for the performance, and exclaim with surprise and (mock?) embarrassment,

"Did I really do that?" They conveniently ignore the fact that they had voluntarily stepped onto the stage.

My own observations have consistently shown that when I inadvertently offered suggestions of which the patients disapproved for any reason, they did not follow the suggestions. A typical example is that of a young woman who was instructed to imagine herself in a nice, quiet, comfortable room watching a television set. Although she was an excellent hypnotic subject who had used hypnosis with me successfully on several prior occasions, she did not follow this suggestion. I asked why not and she responded, "I'd rather be outdoors." The suggestion was changed to, "Imagine yourself in a nice, quiet, comfortable wooded glen watching a television set," and she complied.

Patients who have feared not knowing what would be happening while hypnotized are pleasantly reassured to find they *do* know exactly what is happening the whole time. Because they are completely aware of what is happening, at times they wonder if they were really hypnotized. But, if the patient were not aware of what was going on, how could he follow the directions of the therapist? Even the nonhypnotized sleepwalker must be aware of what he is doing, or he would be bumping into walls, chairs, etc., on his excursions. The victim of temporal lobe seizures must also be aware of what he is doing, or he would be unable to carry out his complicated activities. The sleepwalker and the temporal lobe patient, however, have amnesia for what occurred, and this gives the impression, in retrospect, that they were unaware.

If the hypnotic patient develops amnesia for the trance period, he, too, in retrospect will believe he was unaware of what was happening while hypnotized. If, in an explanation about hypnosis, the patient is told he will remember everything, it is exceedingly rare for him to develop amnesia for the trance period. There is value in telling this to the patient, but one small exception should be added: "If material comes out during the session which I believe might be too disturbing for you to handle at this time, I will suggest you forget it again until such time as you are able to handle it." It is rare for material of such a disturbing nature to come forth,

but if the therapist suspects any hypnotic experience to be too un-
settling, he can offer the aforementioned suggestion. Almost always
the patient can handle it and so he does remember it, but occasionally re-repression does take place. Often such patients later
report that the amnesia lifted in bits and pieces until they were
again comfortably aware of what they had discovered during the
trance.

The patient who fears becoming weak-willed can be reassured
that this will not happen. He quickly learns to appreciate that the
ability to utilize a suggestion is a strength, not a weakness. It is a
strength which enables him to learn more about himself and to
control himself in new and important ways which include the ability
to reject prior, nonhypnotic suggestions which had been having ad-
verse effects upon him.

Those are the major misconceptions usually encountered. Lesser
ones concern the methods of induction. There are innumerable
ways to induce a hypnotic state, but each therapist generally finds
one with which he is comfortable. Perhaps he finds several with
which he is comfortable to be used in those few instances in which
his usual technique does not work well. However, there is seldom
need for more than one technique, except for the therapist who
enjoys displaying his virtuosity.

There are melodramatic techniques; staring piercingly into the
subject's eyes and repeating hypnotic-sounding words works, but the
melodrama is hardly worth the eye fatigue the hypnotist endures.
Swinging a crystal ball in front of the subject's face works with a
nice mystical flair, but the mystique is hardly worth the arm fatigue.
Using strobe lights synchronized to the patient's brain waves works
with a scientific aura, but the equipment is expensive. The showy
techniques are ideal for the stage hypnotist; the serious therapist
does very nicely with simple, quiet inductions.

HYPNOTIZABILITY AND DEPTH OF HYPNOSIS

Before describing actual induction techniques, there are a few
things to be said about tests for hypnotizability and for depth of

hypnosis. Some writers have a great fondness for such tests; I do not. For research purposes, perhaps, such tests are useful, but for clinical purposes the usefulness remains undemonstrated. I use one technique almost exclusively, and after tallying its effectiveness recently, I found that when I applied it to one hundred consecutive patients, ninety-seven went into the hypnotic state on the first attempt. Checking my induction rates over the years, the average has been 94 to 96 percent, which is approximately what other therapists have found.

As far as testing for "depth" is concerned, virtually all of the aforementioned 97 patients obtained a sufficient depth by the second attempt to utilize ideomotor ideation, ego state therapy, or other treatment modalities as indicated. Therapy was not successful in all of them, but there were therapeutic failures in some who appeared to be the most easily hypnotized and who appeared to go most fully into a trance. There were successes among those I would have classed as more difficult inductees. Parenthetically, failures are to be expected in any form of therapy. Nothing works all the time.

For those who do enjoy administering tests, one of the better is the Hypnotic Induction Profile, developed by Spiegel and Spiegel (1978) and well described in their book, *Trance and Treatment.* This book also includes descriptions of and references to a number of other tests, for those who are inclined to use them. For practical purposes, attempting an induction is a sufficient test into itself and generally takes less time than a formal test would take.

Testing for depth of hypnosis seems equally unnecessary for psychotherapeutic activity. The patient who *looks* deeply and thoroughly relaxed may be assumed to have entered a sufficient depth, and such an assumption is rarely wrong.

HYPNOTIC INDUCTION

The following technique is a compilation of many techniques but bears most resemblance to that of the Spiegels. There is no reason to believe it to be any better than other techniques. It is easy, effective, relatively fast, and completely comfortable for both the operator and the subject. The reader might find it helpful to read through the induction once, ignoring the annotations, so as to get the feel and rhythm of it; reading through a second time with the annotations should help explain the rationale.

I prefer working with the patient in a reclining chair, so he will have support for his head and will be in as relaxing a position as possible. I prefer placing my own chair only inches away from his. The reclining chair is nice, if available, but patients can be hypnotized sitting erect or even standing.

(Putting three fingers on the point of the patient's chin, as if holding it gently in place.[1]) "Keep your head still, but roll your eyeballs as far as you can toward the back of your head.[2] You may feel your eyes becoming strained,[3] but this will last only a few more moments." (Remove your fingers from the chin.) "Now, while you're still looking upward, slowly close your eyes.[4] Take a deep breath; good; let it out, and now let your eye muscles relax. Notice the rapid fluttering of your eyelids;[5] that is one of the first signs of entering the hypnotic state.[6] As you go more deeply into it, the fluttering will stop.[7]

"Now, let yourself imagine what it might feel like to be floating,[8] floating any way you like—floating downward, softly, like a feather; or floating upward, gently like a balloon; or floating evenly, like a leaf upon a pond.[9] As you imagine what it feels like to be floating, perhaps you'll notice . . . you're becoming more and more relaxed with every breath.[10] While you're becoming more and more relaxed with every breath,[11] I'll be working with your right arm.[12]

"First, I'm going to touch it lightly with one fingertip." (Do so, running the finger gently from the hand up to the elbow.) "Now, even though I'm no longer touching the arm,[13] you'll still be able to feel the light trace of my finger on it.[14] The light trace will seem to spread throughout the arm. The arm will seem to grow lighter and lighter. The arm will grow so light it will begin to rise off the arm of the chair, right up toward the ceiling. Good, you can feel the arm beginning to rise.[15] You're doing beautifully.[16] Right on up, higher and higher, lighter and lighter, moving automatically, as if it had a life of its own.[17] It may be a slightly strange sensation, but it will be pleasant.[18]

"Now, without coming out of your hypnotic state,[19] when I count to three let your eyes open[20] so you can watch that hand as it continues to rise.[21] That's fine, it will stop there" (touching the back of the hand) "and will remain right there, easily and effortlessly until I snap my fingers. When I snap my fingers, the arm will become so heavy it can no longer stay up.[22] As it sinks to the chair again, your eyelids will become heavy and sleepy, they will close, and you will feel yourself sinking into one of the most pleasant, relaxing states you have enjoyed in a long, long while." (Move your fingers slowly into the patient's visual field, then snap them.) "Good, now just let yourself go into it more and more deeply.[23] The deeper you go, the more comfortable you become."

Discussion

Without reading any further, the average person could repeat something similar to what has just been described and probably find he could induce a hypnotic state in 90 to 95 percent of willing subjects. Anyone just starting to practice this, however, should realize the exact words are much less important than a feeling of comfort when saying them. Rehearsal into a tape recorder will speed up this acquisition of comfort, but nothing produces a sense of confidence like success with a few subjects. Incidentally, one's own spouse is frequently a resistant subject, for reasons that are easy to imagine, so the beginner should look elsewhere for his or her early attempts.

The following annotations may help explain the rationale for the steps described. They also offer an opportunity to include certain miscellaneous thoughts and data.

[1] When most patients are asked to roll their eyeballs backward, they also tend to roll their heads backward, putting their necks in an uncomfortable position. Holding the chin prevents this from happening and also gives the nonverbal clue that the hypnotist is beginning to take charge.

[2] Elman (1964) is the first writer of whom I am aware to

specifically note that straining the muscles of the eye enhances entry into the hypnotic state; he used a lateral gaze. The old eye-fixation methods of induction, however, also employed this principle by having the subject look at an object above his forehead.

[3] The eye muscles become strained as a physiological response to looking up so high, but commenting on the strain reassures the patient that the operator knows what is happening to him and/or may lead the patient to see the strain as an effect that is being produced by the hypnosis. To know he is experiencing what he is supposed to experience is a further reassurance to the patient.

[4] Most subjects feel more relaxed with the eyelids closed, but having the subject close his eyes while still gazing upward allows the operator to measure the "eye-roll sign," the amount of sclera that is visible between the lower lid and the lower border of the iris. This sign, described by the Spiegels, is part of their Hypnotic Induction Profile and is hypothesized by them to be a measurement of the inherent ability of the subject to be hypnotized.

[5] Do not say this unless the eyelids *are* fluttering rapidly. They almost always do, and this is thought to be one of the physiological occurrences in the hypnotic state. There are others, none of them invariably constant. The sclera frequently become injected, lacrimation may occur without any feelings of sadness, and the palms may become warm and moist. The fluttering, injection of the sclera, and lacrimation could all be caused by the induced eyestrain, but they also may occur when other induction techniques are used.

[6] This is both a reassurance about the fluttering and a further suggestion that the subject is becoming hypnotized.

[7] The fluttering always does stop, although it may recur throughout most of the induction. When it does stop, the patient will already have been told this means he has entered a deeper state of hypnosis, and this suggestion will help him do so.

[8] Do not use this suggestion with a patient who has been complaining of feelings of depersonalization, as if his feet were not touching the ground; he may find it uncomfortable. Instead, have him imagine any other feeling which he might find relaxing. The use of imagination seems to enhance the hypnotic effect; Kroger

and Fezler (1976) have written extensively describing their systematic use of it.

[9] It's unnecessary to offer a wide variety of floating experiences, but the repetitive descriptions of a pleasant experience are soothing. Different patients will select different ones of these images, or at times will invent ones of their own. Although invention of his own image instead of accepting the one offered by the hypnotist could be viewed as a resistance to the suggestion, in my experience the inventive patient is generally a superior subject, and so these inventions are always appreciated.

[10] "Perhaps you'll notice . . . you're becoming more relaxed." The perhaps gives leeway to both the subject and the operator in case the subject is not yet becoming more relaxed. Equally importantly, the whole phrase suggests the patient should become aware of something that is already happening, but he may not have noticed it yet.

The above is a crude example of the style Milton Erickson used so brilliantly in his work with hypnosis. Erickson was considered by many the foremost clinical hypnotist in America, but his methods were so incredibly clever that few therapists could ever duplicate them. I suspect a great many beginners have been discouraged in their attempts to do so, and anyone without his unique talents would do far better to learn more simplified approaches. A careful analysis of Erickson's techniques has been presented by Bandler and Grinder (1973); this makes his approach more understandable but still very difficult to emulate.

[11] Another Ericksonian-like comment—an explicit expectation that the subject *is* becoming more relaxed.

[12] Or the left arm, depending upon where the operator is sitting in relation to the patient. It is conceivable one may be better than the other because of the lateralized functions of the human brain, but at this time there is insufficient evidence to justify rearranging the furniture in the room.

[13] Take your finger off first.

[14] This normal physiological response, more prominent in subjects with hairy arms, is usually interpreted by the subject as a result of the hypnotic suggestion. Each time a subject believes he

is responding hypnotically, there seems to be increasing ease for further responding.

[15] Obviously, this should not be said unless the arm *is* beginning to rise. If the arm is not yet beginning to do so, without breaking cadence the operator may say, "I'll help it a little to begin with. I'll take your wrist and help it start." He gently takes hold of the wrist and, using the lightest pressure necessary to encourage the arm upward, looks for slight, jerky muscular contractions that soon begin to raise the arm on its own. He should make comment on those contractions as well as on the fact that he is now using less pressure to lift the arm. Once the arm is moving well on its own, he may say, "Now that it is moving by itself, I will remove my fingers and the arm will continue to rise."

[16] Everyone likes praise, but the hypnotic subject, uncertain of his ability to be hypnotized, is further relaxed by this comment on his success.

[17] This encourages a sense of dissociation between the subject and his arm and enhances the notion that he is not merely being cooperative in lifting his arm to please the therapist.

[18] It does feel pleasant, and it does feel slightly strange. Again, the patient is reassured by letting him know the operator is aware of what he is experiencing, and simultaneously the patient is encouraged by letting him know he is having the "proper" response.

[19] Suggesting, of course, that he is already in a hypnotic state.

[20] A subtle suggestion that the eyes will open when the operator counts to three if only the patient permits them to do so.

[21] Having visible or other evidence of behaving in response to hypnotic suggestion seems to deepen the level of hypnosis.

[22] This incorporates the "reverse arm levitation" technique as part of the induction and permits the patient to witness more of his responding to suggestion. "It can no longer stay up" adds to the dissociative feeling and avoids a direct confrontation with the patient as would occur with, "You can no longer hold it up."

[23] Subjectively, "deeper" means feeling more relaxed. There have already been comments about measuring the depth of hypnosis, which I consider unnecessary since virtually any subject who *looks*

well relaxed is capable of following the suggestions used in the techniques for doing psychotherapy via hypnosis.

This has been a long explanation of the induction process which is actually brief and simple. Just as it is unnecessary to memorize the induction, likewise it is unnecessary to learn all the annotations. A basic rationale for what the operator is doing and a feel for what is happening are far more important than any specifics.

OTHER INDUCTION TECHNIQUES

Since the percentage of patients responding to the above technique approximates the percentage of patients who are capable of responding at all, there is seldom need for other methods, but there are a few instances in which variations can prove useful.

The briefest variation is to say one word, "Sleep." If the patient has come to the office already believing the therapist is an accomplished hypnotist, expecting to be hypnotized, and has started displaying a faraway, dreamy look on his face during the explanations about hypnosis, this technique will work almost every time, although occasionally the word will need to be repeated once or twice.

A rare patient will express or display fear about keeping his eyes closed. If a brief discussion of his fear does not dispel it, the following variation may be used: "Open your eyes as wide as you can and look up as high as you can." (This will initiate eyestrain, as in the original technique described, will acknowledge his fear, and will utilize his wish as part of the induction.) "Now, without moving your head, watch your right hand as closely as possible." (This continues eyestrain, but in a downward direction.) "I'm going to stroke your hand and arm lightly with one fingertip. . . ." (Continue the original technique to the point of snapping the fingers to make the arm become heavy but change the suggestion from the one including the eyes closing to:) "When I snap my fingers, your arm will become so heavy it will no longer stay up. As it sinks, you will feel yourself becoming more and more relaxed, going deeper and deeper into the hypnotic state. As you become more relaxed, you may wish to close your eyes" (giving him permission to do so, rather than a command), "but I *want* you to open them again whenever you choose!" (implying that they will close, and that if he does open them again, this is in response to a command.)

This technique will induce eye closure most of the time, but it is important to note that there is no absolute need for the hypnotized patient to have his eyes closed. The therapist and the patient both *feel* more convinced the induction has worked if eye closure has occurred, but this arises primarily from tradition and from our falsely associating hypnosis with sleep. The somnambulistic state of hypnosis, one of the deepest obtainable, permits the patient to walk with his eyes open, talk, and behave in almost every other way as if he were not hypnotized, and yet he will respond to any acceptable command the hypnotist offers.

Another rare occurrence is the patient who becomes frightened whenever he begins to relax, so naturally it would be unwise to begin an induction with the soothing, relaxing suggestions of the first technique. A variation might be (all of this said with an authoritarian voice): "Sit down! Put your hands together and intertwine your fingers. Lock them together as tightly as you can. Watch them closely. Squeeze them together so tightly they begin to hurt. Watch the knuckles turn white as you squeeze them harder and harder. They're beginning to feel locked together, fused together, welded together—so solidly welded together they can't come apart. Even when they try, they can't come apart." (Note the use of "they can't come apart" rather than "you can't pull them apart.") "Good. Now they're relaxing. Close your eyes. Close them as tightly as you can. So tightly they feel stuck together, so tight they can't come apart even if they try. Good. Now that the hypnosis is taking control, it's safe for you to begin relaxing."

This type of patient is almost always afraid of relaxing because he is afraid of losing control of himself in one way or another. It will become a primary function of therapy to discover the origin of the fear and alleviate it, but once he feels the therapist is in control, he becomes able to lower his defensive posture.

A less rare patient is the one who says he wishes to be hypnotized but displays a variety of resistances. These may take the form of asking questions during the induction, shifting his posture frequently, laughing, or actively (though subtly) pushing his arm downward as the therapist attempts to raise it.

If the patient interrupts with questions, the therapist might say, "Questions frequently arise during the induction, and I'll be pleased to answer them in a few minutes. Do not ask them now, just let yourself be more and more aware of what you're experiencing, and perhaps you'll find the answers for yourself."

In response to smiling, laughing, moving, etc., the therapist might say, "I want you to be as comfortable as possible, so I want you to smile, move, scratch your nose, or do anything that will make you more comfortable and allow you to go deeper into the hypnotic state." (Here there are the implications the movements are the suggestions of the therapist and that they will enhance the induction.)

If there are more active resistances, I will use the original technique described but will schedule several brief sessions, ending each by saying, "Now that you see what we're trying to do, you'll feel more comfortable with it, and the next time we work together perhaps you'll find it easier to experience what I'm suggesting."

There are other techniques for dealing with the resistant patient: confusion techniques, arm rotation or other repetitive arm movements, the incredibly subtle methods of Erickson, etc., but frankly, if the methods described above don't work for me, the other techniques don't work either, so I'll not describe them here.

There is another form of resistance that should be mentioned—the patient who has been hypnotized but doubts or denies that he was. I know of no way to prove to a person that he has been hypnotized, and if he is challenged with, "How do you explain this or that happening?" he will either offer a rationalization or say, "I can't explain it, but I know I wasn't hypnotized." The therapist can ask this patient, "Did you feel really relaxed?" and if he concedes he did, the therapist can say, "Good. I know you could fake your arm going up or down, or fake not being able to open your eyes, but you can't fake a feeling; either you have it or you don't. If you felt really relaxed, that's good enough. Perhaps it's not really hypnosis, but if you can get that good, relaxed feeling, you'll be able to do what we want to do." And usually he can.

ENDING THE HYPNOTIC STATE

Once the trance is induced, the beginning hypnotherapist often wonders, "What do I do next?" There are innumerable things that can be done, not the least of which is ending the trance. This is even easier than inducing it, and there are countless ways to do so, but one simple technique will suffice, except for those rare patients who do not respond. Helping them out of the trance was discussed previously.

A subject who is startled out of his trance may feel a little uncomfortable briefly, as though he had been startled out of a nap. To avoid creating that discomfort, the operator should avoid suggestions like, "You'll awaken when I clap my hands." More considerate would be, "In a moment I will count backward from three. As I do, you'll awaken with a remarkably pleasant feeling of relaxation that will stay with you for a long while afterwards. Three . . . two . . . one . . . zero . . . awaken." Patients later report they maintained the comfortable feeling anywhere from a few minutes to a few days.

REINDUCTION OF THE HYPNOTIC STATE

If the therapist will be hypnotizing the patient a second time or many times, he may use the same induction technique he used originally, but considerable time can be saved by use of a post-hypnotic suggestion during the first trance. The post-hypnotic suggestion may be virtually anything the hypnotist chooses, as long as it does not offend the patient. Examples would be: "You will reenter the hypnotic state when I . . . (snap my fingers three times, or rap my desk twice with this cigarette lighter)." Although either of these would work for the majority of patients, I feel it is a little demeaning to the patient to make such a blunt demand. I prefer something like, "In the future, to use our time more effectively, you will be *able* to reenter the hypnotic state quickly, deeply, and pleasantly when I ask you to look upward for a few seconds and when I say the word 'sleep.' " I generally add, "You will never enter the hypnotic state accidentally or unless you're willing to do so." The addition is useful, for before adding it, I did have a few patients go into the state unintentionally.

The post-hypnotic suggestions for reinduction are useful primarily for reinductions that will occur at future appointments. If the patient is to be rehypnotized within minutes after being brought out of his first trance, he may be asked how he is feeling, be given an opportunity to ask any questions which may have arisen, and then told, "You were a very good hypnotic subject, and now you will be pleased to find you can reenter the trance easily and pleasantly when I . . . (squeeze your wrist, or pass my hand before your face, or whatever the therapist chooses)."

Teaching the Subject Self-hypnosis

This is surprisingly easy to do, and although it can be presented as a long, drawn-out series of sessions, there is no reason for doing so except the unscrupulous rewards derived from presenting it as a long, drawn-out series of sessions. Just as a simple, post-hypnotic suggestion enables the therapist to reinduce the hypnotic state, in the same way a simple post-hypnotic suggestion will enable the subject to reenter the trance without any help from the hypnotist.

"From this time on, whenever you wish to hypnotize yourself, all you need do is. . . ." Again, any ritual will work. I use, "Strain your eyes upward for about five seconds, then slowly spell the word R-E-L-A-X." Straining the eyes, as mentioned previously, seems to facilitate entry into a trance state, and "relax" is a direct suggestion for what is expected to happen.

Patients may express concern about being able to bring themselves out of the state but they can be reassured the post-hypnotic suggestion for awakening will be just as effective as the one for the induction. "Whenever you wish to come out of it, all you need do is count backwards from three and open your eyes. Upon coming out of it, you will be alert and well-coordinated and will feel more relaxed for a long while after."

I then have the patient practice self-hypnosis while still in the office. I have him practice while reclined in the chair, while sitting erect in a less comfortable chair, and while standing up. The repeated practice is useful, the idea that he need not be recumbent for it to work is useful, and the ability to hypnotize himself while standing up is very practical. Patients who are at work or at a party may stand up, pretend to be reading a bulletin board or looking out the window, and relax themselves without anyone else being aware of what they are doing.

Apparently, the only danger in doing self-hypnosis is the possibility of falling asleep, and that is dangerous only if the patient has an appointment to keep. Once sleep sets in, the hypnosis is apparently ended and anything which would ordinarily awaken the patient will awaken him. If, during the self-imposed trance, some emergency arises, the patient will be totally aware of the emergency and will emerge from the trance without the formality of counting backward.

Reportedly, there is one other danger of self-hypnosis; the patient may become "addicted" to hypnosis. The one patient of mine in whom this happened was a creative young lady who started spending inordinate amounts of her free time in a fantasy world she conjured while in a self-imposed trance. This went on for a couple of months; she then grew tired of it and began writing a book based upon the fantasies.

A RECOMMENDATION

Although the techniques described above are easily learned merely by reading and practicing them, there are definite advantages to taking formal courses from skilled instructors. Observing others using these or similar techniques and practicing them under supervision are very helpful in polishing one's style, generating a greater feeling of confidence, and correcting any mistakes which might appear.

Nationally, there are two excellent professional societies which offer courses for beginners or advanced students: the American

Society of Clinical Hypnosis and the Society of Clinical and Experimental Hypnosis. Locally, at least in larger communities, there may be affiliate branches of one or the other of these organizations. Additionally, individuals, groups of individuals, and a number of universities offer courses well worth the time and effort.

AN ADDITIONAL RECOMMENDATION

Although the hypnotic techniques themselves are simple, no attempt at doing therapeutic work via hypnosis should be undertaken by anyone not formally trained in doing therapeutic work via more conventional means. Learning how to do hypnosis, in some respects, is comparable to learning how to give an injection. The process is easily acquired by anyone with moderate intelligence, but there is potential for serious harm unless the person giving the injection has been well trained as to what medication should be put into the syringe, in what doses, and for what conditions. He should also be trained in how to handle any unexpected side effects from the medication injected.

CHAPTER FOUR

Uncovering Techniques

❖❖❖❖❖❖❖❖❖❖❖❖❖❖❖❖❖❖❖❖❖❖❖❖❖❖❖❖❖❖ ❖❖❖❖❖❖❖❖❖❖❖❖❖❖❖❖❖❖❖❖

Throughout the years a number of different techniques have been devised to aid in the recovery of repressed material and the attendant affects. It is easy to describe the techniques; it is difficult, if not impossible, to offer clear explanations of how or why they work. They do work, however, and there is no need to deny patients the benefits of their efficacy until the theorists have evolved suitable explanations.

Many of the techniques which have been around for years still have merit, but none has the efficacy of the three to be described in the second part of this chapter—ideomotor responding, the affect bridge, and ego state therapy. The lesser ones will be mentioned briefly; the major ones will receive considerably more attention, with case illustrations to give a fuller flavor of what occurs.

MINOR UNCOVERING TECHNIQUES

Relaxation

The hypnotized patient almost invariably is more relaxed than
the nonhypnotized patient. The relaxed patient is less defensive
than the nonrelaxed patient. Therefore, merely inducing a state of
relaxation permits the patient to free associate and elaborate on his
associations more easily than he might do otherwise. For a thoughtful and well-documented description of analytic work combined
with hypnosis, Brenman and Gill's *Hypnotherapy* (1971) is highly
recommended.

An interesting and sometimes minor variation of doing insight-
oriented work in the office is to teach the patient self-hypnosis and
have him spend small amounts of time at home in a self-induced
trance asking one simple question repeatedly, "Why should this
feeling still be here?" or "What does it really mean when I . . .?" etc.
Very interesting and informative answers sometimes appear, giving
rich material to be explored at the next session.

Dreams

The post-hypnotic suggestion, "Tonight you will have a dream
or series of dreams which will help give us a clearer understanding
of . . ." will often produce dreams that indeed help give a clearer
understanding. There is no good evidence, though, that hypnosis
used in this manner is more effective than the more subtle suggestions therapists gave without hypnosis, "We will examine your
dreams and your fantasies, too, so report them as part of the work we
will be doing."

If a reported dream is vague or incomplete, however, hypnosis
may be used to have the patient redream the dream in the office,
thus obtaining greater clarity or completeness. When this is done,
two legitimate and perhaps unanswerable questions can arise: Is
the redreamed dream the same as the original one, and how much
difference does it really make? The dream produced in the office

could be at least as important as the original one since it, too, should be the product of unconscious thought processes.

If a patient presents a dream but offers no useful associations to it, hypnosis can be used to suggest the patient relax and let associations come to him. This combination of relaxation and direct suggestion may raise questions regarding the validity of the interpretations the patient then makes, but how different is it from the direct, nonhypnotic suggestion, "Tell me whatever thoughts come to mind?" There may be at least two differences: 1) The hypnotic suggestion, by producing more relaxation, could be more effective, and 2) the patient may have less sense of being an active participant in the therapy.

Fantasies

Closely related to the dreamwork described above is the hypnotic suggestion that the patient will permit himself to have a fantasy about whatever material is being discussed. A more complicated ritual would be for the therapist to guide the patient on a fantasy to some given point and let the patient take over from there. "You are walking through this old, empty house you lived in when you were a child and you come to a locked door. You try to open the door but cannot find the key. You pound the door with your fists, then kick it again and again until the rusty lock gives way. You open the door and peer inside. Look around carefully and describe what you are seeing."

Automatic Writing

Some hypnotic subjects can be taught to write, apparently without conscious knowledge of what they are writing, while they are simultaneously talking to the therapist or engaged in some other activity. If the therapist has suggested a topic for the writing, unconscious material on that topic will be produced, but most patients require extensive training before they are able to do this, and there are easier methods for obtaining the same data (or what are presumed to be the same data).

Hypnoplasty, Hypnography

These techniques are essentially the same as automatic writing, but instead of producing written words, the subjects produce sculptured or drawn images. I suppose there could also be hypnodancing, hypnomiming or hypnoanything the therapist has some particular interest in, as long as the patient is willing to go along with it.

"Seeing" a Movie, TV, Play, etc.

(With elaboration) "You are sitting in the theatre now, and the movie begins. It is a movie about you when you were nine years old and you were told your parents were getting a divorce. As you watch this movie of what happened then, tell me what you are seeing." This is a more detached and depersonalized variation of age regression which is useful if the therapist and/or patient believes actual age regression could produce too strong a negative affect.

Age Regression

"You are on a train going backward in time. As I count from ten down to one, with each number you go back a few more years. When I reach one, you will be back to your seventh birthday party. You will see all your friends who were there and you will see all the presents you received. And then something happens that gets you upset."

At times this technique will not produce an "age regression" but will merely evoke a remembrance of the scene. The patient will say, "I was talking to Kathy when my brother came up and told her I wet the bed last night." Details might follow, but there may be little affect connected to it. If the regression is more successful, it will be, "I'm talking to Kathy . . .," with the material being recounted in the present tense, voice and vocabulary being more consonant with a seven-year-old's, and considerable affect being displayed. This technique and variations of it are most useful when combined with other techniques. Many therapists recommend "practice" age regressions to pleasant periods in the patient's life before trying a regression to a traumatic incident.

Major Uncovering Techniques

Far superior to any of the above are ideomotor responding, the affect bridge, and ego state therapy. They enable the patient to move rapidly to the dynamics that underlie his problems. They lead to those dynamics without the meanderings of free association. They lead there without the intellectually stimulating but intermittent successes of dream interpretation. They lead there without the prolonged process of analysis of defenses.

Many of us were taught that if the defenses are not analyzed there can be no basic change in the personality. Experience does not support this thesis. The defenses, after all, did not grow out of thin air to plague us; they were erected specifically to defend against the revelation of past experiences, impulses, and affects. Once those experiences, impulses, and/or affects are exposed and assimilated, the defenses are no longer needed and quietly wither away.

The origin of the defense is stated more masterfully by Greenson (1967, p. 80):

> The immediate cause is always the avoidance of some painful affect like anxiety, guilt or shame. The more distal cause is the underlying instinctual impulse which stirred up the anxiety, guilt or shame. The ultimate cause is the traumatic situation, a state in which the ego is overwhelmed and helpless because it is flooded with anxiety it cannot control, master, or bind—a state of panic.

The disappearance of the defense is stated masterfully by Dewald (1972, p. 625):

> As a result of the gradual dissolution of the danger situation through application of secondary process reasoning, and the concomitant reduction of the painful associated affects, the previously unconscious needs for specifically structured and automatic defensive responses to such situations is likewise reduced.

Further comments about defenses may be useful at this point. As we know, the more comfortable the patient feels with his therapist, the less defensive he will be. All of us have had the experience of dealing with *conscious* defenses when the patient says, "I don't know if I can tell you this yet." We ask what is preventing his telling us and we hear, "I don't know if I can trust you," or "I'm afraid you'll think I'm terrible." *Unconscious* defenses, based upon similar fears arising from unconscious transference feelings about the therapist, will also prevent revelations, perhaps as much to protect the patient from the critical judgment of the therapist as to protect him from his own critical judgment.

Sometimes, however, protection from the therapist is more of a reality issue than we like to admit. First, even though we attempt to maintain a neutral stance, I am convinced we display more positive or negative affect than we believe we do. The display may be subtle—inflections in the tone of voice or slight shifts in our bodily postures—but the patient, expecting the reprimands or praise, will often be exquisitely attuned to our signals.

Next, the manner in which interpretation is sometimes made can justifiably be classified as an accusation. For example, "So, despite the tender hugs and kisses you gave him, it sounds as though you really hated your teddy bear." The interpretation may be absolutely correct, but the patient may meet it with stout resistance because the therapist is accusing him of being both hateful and deceitful. If, on the other hand, the interpretation has been, "So, despite the tender hugs and kisses you gave him, it sounds as though you really hated your teddy bear *because your brother beat you over the head with it*," there would no longer be an accusation, there would be an explanation which justified the hate and which converted the deceit into ambivalence. Resistance to this interpretation would be unnecessary.

We all presume we make our interpretations in the most helpful way. These presumptions may be erroneous. Many times patients have told me, "It's a relief to talk to you about this. My former therapist (s) always made me feel guilty when I told him (them) anything about myself." I expect other therapists have heard the same about me.

The hypnotic state is such a relaxing state in itself that resistances are already lowered, as was mentioned previously. I believe there are two other factors which also tend to diminish resistance when the following uncovering techniques are used.

1) The repressed material is recovered in the full context of what was happening to the patient at the time of repression, so the explanation for the repressed action or feeling is more readily apparent.

2) There seems to be a partial splitting of the patient's ego into an adult, self-observing ego and a younger, experiencing ego. This splitting, or perhaps partial dissociation, allows the self-observing portion to comprehend what happened without the full impact of the affect. The other portion appears capable of handling the full impact, albeit with varying degrees of discomfort.

When hypnotic techniques are used, patients do not suffer embarrassing "confessions" as they often do in more conventional therapy; they join in exciting explorations of their past life.

IDEOMOTOR RESPONDING

Ideomotor responding is one of the three major techniques for uncovering dynamics and attendant affect. Ideo refers to ideas and motor refers to motor muscles which can be utilized to evoke movement in response to certain ideas. When the responses are elicited properly, it is believed they come from unconscious sources, and clinical experience tends to support this belief. Patients can readily understand the concept of unconscious ideas causing motor muscles to move: "Have you ever had the experience of someone asking, 'Why are you frowning?' and you didn't realize you were frowning?" (The answer is almost invariably yes.) "Well, that means something you weren't aware of was bothering you, and that caused the muscles of your face to move into a frown." Therapists should be even more aware of this phenomenon than patients, for they are accustomed to observing body language and commenting on it to help the patient become more aware of unconscious feelings.

Once the patient understands this part of the concept, it is easy to explain that we can use hypnosis to get specific muscles moving in response to specific questions. Generally, I suggest the index finger move to signal "yes," the middle finger move to signal "no," and both fingers move to signal "I don't want to answer that question." The last signal is partly superfluous because the patient wouldn't answer the question if he didn't want to, but I add it to reassure him that it is permissible to keep secrets if he chooses to do so.

Some therapists do not specify which finger will give the affirmative answer and which the negative one, letting the patient choose his own signals. They may also add an additional signal for a response meaning, "I don't know the answer." This seems to be a matter of personal preference for the therapist; patients do well with the signals I first mentioned.

Before proceeding with a description of how ideomotor responding is used clinically, I will first mention the seven basic psychodynamics of Leslie LeCron, for combining the use of those seven dynamics with the ideomotor responses can give the therapist a better idea of the directions in which he and the patient may end up moving. LeCron's book, *The Complete Guide to Hypnosis* (1971), although far less complete than the title would indicate, still remains a useful reference work and describes the seven dynamics and the ideomotor responding (or the use of a chevreul pendulum) in greater detail than I will offer here. I have rearranged his order of listing the dynamics and paraphrased some of them to aid in my own conceptualization of what they mean.

1) *Body Language.* Many symptoms, particularly the psychophysiological ones, appear to be symbolic expressions of feelings the patient is unable to express in a more direct manner, usually not even to himself. For examples, torticollis, in which the neck remains pulled painfully to one side, may be expressing, "I can't stand to look at what lies ahead." Chronic diarrhea could be, "I can't stomach any more of this crap."

2) *Imprint.* Imprinting refers to the process whereby concepts are strongly implanted into the patient's patterns of thinking or feeling. Patterns of behavior and self-concepts can be the direct result of what the patient was told. He begins to believe what he

was told and then causes it to become true. A typical example would be, "You're a lazy, stupid kid, and you'll never be worth a damn." To be imprinted, the message must be repeated frequently enough to make its impact, or it may be said only once, during a period of strong emotional experience. Not infrequently, patients refer to this phenomenon spontaneously: "I can't seem to erase the old tapes my parents put in my head saying I was lazy and no-good and would never amount to anything."

One of the more interesting cases which I believe illustrates imprinting, both in the origin of symptoms and the cure of them, occurred in a young man in group therapy, with no hypnosis involved. From childhood on, he had received negative comments about himself almost identical to the examples given above. He had believed the comments and had conducted his life in accord with the dire predictions made. In a severe depression he became drunk, took an overdose of sleeping pills and fell down, lacerating his head. He was discovered and taken to the hospital; while there, in the emotional state following his close brush with death, he had visits from friends who spoke of his positive qualities and their belief in his ability to lead a successful life. His life started becoming successful from that point on.

3) *Past Experience.* This is rather similar to imprinting but results from an actual experience or series of experiences rather than from something the patient had been told. Having had the experience, the patient anticipates that similar situations will produce similar results. He therefore reacts to new situations with old behavioral patterns and old, inappropriate affects. Needless to say, his responses frequently are not in his own best interests. Almost all phobias can be linked directly to a specific past experience; this statement, which does not coincide with certain analytic concepts, will receive further elaboration later. Also, the reader may have noted the similarity between transference reactions and the effects of the past experience.

4) *Secondary Gain.* This dynamic should be familiar to almost anyone who has worked with patients. It simply means the symptom, no matter how unpleasant, offers the patient a reward for his

having the symptom. The reward is almost never sufficient to repay the patient for the suffering the symptom causes, and at times there is no reward at all, only the hope of a reward. The patient, for example, who unconsciously believes his illness will bring sympathy and understanding may find he is treated with irritation and neglect. His unconscious, however, operating in the illogical ways the unconscious seems to operate, may futilely continue to produce the symptom in the vain hope of receiving the reward.

5) *Identification.* A patient may manifest a symptom as the result of an unconscious identification with some important person who had the same or similar symptom. The important person is usually a member of the patient's family but can be a fictional character from a book, play, opera, etc., that had an important meaning for him.

6) *Conflict.* This has the traditional meaning; i.e., the patient has a wish for something which is prohibited by his parents, society, or his own inner feelings. The symptom either prevents carrying out the wish or is a symbolic fulfillment of the wish. An example of the preventive aspect was found in one patient whose "paralysis" of her lower extremities prevented her from acting on the wish to assault her sister. An example of the symbolic aspect was found in a patient whose continued plucking of her pubic hairs was derived from her masturbatory impulses.

7) *Self-punishment.* Not infrequently a symptom serves primarily as a means of punishing the patient for some long-forgotten sin. Theoretically, this has been said to occur either to relieve guilty feelings or to avoid harsher punishment from some higher authority. In actual practice it seems to occur more frequently as a harsh and continuing example of what will happen if the patient "sins" again. Almost always the sin is of minor import, and it is a cruel irony that patients who commit real atrocities are less likely to be troubled by pangs of conscience than patients who commit minor violations of the codes of their superegos. This does not seem to be true in veterans of Viet Nam who had terrible guilt about the atrocities they may have committed, but that war provided a highly atypical environment.

An interesting example of self-punishment was found in a patient who sought hypnosis to help her lose weight. Ideomotor responding revealed her overeating was a means of punishing herself, and the sin was her having stolen a small item from a department store when she was a child. She returned the next week to tell me that all her life she had felt like a liar and a cheat and had never believed any decent person could love her. She had purchased a one dollar money order and mailed it anonymously to the store and was feeling good about herself for the first time in her memory. *Brief Encounters* by Karl Lewin (1970) does not deal with hypnosis but does describe in great detail one method of doing short-term psychotherapy primarily by looking at the self-punishing aspects of the patient's symptoms.

The thoughtful reader will readily see how a symptom could be attributed to several of these seven dynamics simultaneously. For instance, there could have been an event like trying to stuff a baby brother down the toilet (past experience); the parents may have yelled, "You're a horrible, vicious little kid and no one will ever love you" (imprint, said only once but during a highly emotional period); the patient may still want to get rid of that baby brother (conflict), and develop a tic (symbolic stuffing) or a paralysis (prevention of the suffering). The paralysis could be to prevent the stuffing or could be a self-punishment for his past behavior or his current wish. Even though all those factors could be present simultaneously, usually one or two would have much greater significance than the others.

Using ideomotor responding becomes much like playing "Twenty Questions," but with more serious intent. It can best be described by giving an example of its use.

With this, as with all the other uncovering techniques, work is done more effectively if the therapist has listened carefully to the presenting complaints and has obtained at least a brief history from the patient. The listening not only provides valuable information, but also helps establish rapport, which makes the ensuing work easier. The history-taking need not be a prolonged affair; often one session will suffice, and more than two is rarely necessary.

After the history-taking, the therapist can introduce the topic of hypnosis, attend to any concerns about its use, and attempt to answer any questions the patient has. He may get into the ideomotor responses in that same session or he may merely induce a trance once or twice, teach the patient self-hypnosis, and have the patient practice self-hypnosis at home during the week prior to the next session, when the actual uncovering work will begin. Practice prior to starting therapy is not essential.

I prefer explaining ideomotor responding and the seven dynamics before inducing the trance state, but I have also given the explanations while the patient is in trance and have also done the work without explaining the seven dynamics to the patient at all. The outcomes seem to be similar any way it is done, but I feel my task is made easier by the prior explanations. Once the hypnotic state is induced, the session may proceed along lines similar to the one below. This will not be a verbatim transcript of an interview, for there is no need to suffer through all the negative responses that are invariably obtained. The fact that negative responses are frequently obtained is important, however, for it demonstrates the patient does not give only the answers the therapist wishes to receive.

T. Now I shall count backwards from ten. By the time I reach zero, you will be so deeply into the hypnosis it will be possible for me to ask questions of the unconscious and for the unconscious to respond through your fingers. If the answer to my question is "yes," this finger will move up and then down like this (the therapist moves the patient's finger). If the answer is "no," this finger will move up and then down. If for any reason the unconscious does not wish to answer the question, both fingers will move up, then down. Do not *make* your fingers move, just think of the question instead of the answer, and *let* the fingers move.

Ten, nine, . . . zero. We will begin now. Does the unconscious understand my instructions? (Saying the "unconscious" rather than "you" helps add to a feeling of dissociation.)

P. Yes.

T. Good. Does it have any objections to my asking questions in
   this manner? (This gives the therapist and the patient an opportunity to see if both the yes and no answers can be
   obtained.)

P. No.

T. Does this symptom(s) come from one *or more* of the seven dynamics I explained? (The unconscious can respond with great
   concreteness, so if the question were, "Did it come from one
   of the seven dynamics," the answer might be "no" because it
   came from two of them.)

P. Yes.

T. From two or more?

P. Yes.

T. Three or more?

P. No (meaning it came from two).

T. Is one of these much more important than the other one?

P. Yes.

T. Is the most important one an imprint?

P. No.

T. Is the most important one self-punishment?

P. Yes.

T. Are you punishing yourself for something that happened before
   you were twenty years old?

P. Yes.

T. Before you were ten years old? (The therapist continues nar-
   rowing down to a specific age, or if there was a series of events,
   to a specific period in the patient's life.)

T. Is this punishment for something you did?

P. Yes. (If no, the therapist asks, "For something you wished?" or
   "For something you said?")

T. Did you do this to someone else?

P. Yes.

T. Did you do it to a member of your family? (The therapist continues with questions to discover who was the victim, when
   and where the incident(s) occurred, etc.)

Utilizing this type of questioning, it is not unusual to pinpoint the event within fifteen to thirty minutes. Details may include the age of the patient at the time, the time of day, the room of the house in which it occurred, other people present at the time, etc. Even more details can be elicited if the therapist chooses to do so, but considerable time may be saved by pausing at that point to ask the patient, "Is the event present now in the *conscious* mind?"

If the patient answers affirmatively, the therapist can ask, "Are you willing to tell me about it?" If so, then, "Without awakening from your hypnotic state, you can now talk to me with your usual voice and tell me what happened."

If the event is not yet consciously recalled, the therapist could ask, still using ideomotor responses, "Would you be willing to use age regression to go back to the event and live through it again?" If an affirmative answer is received, "Would it be safe for you to do so at this time?" If yes, an age regression technique would then be used.

If the age regression worked, the patient would appear to be experiencing the event again, with changes in his posture and his voice expressing whatever emotions were present originally. In that one session, he would have uncovered the repressed material and the repressed affect. He would have reexperienced the affect to some degree, and the affect would have been attenuated by the reexperiencing and by the conscious recall which would have permitted secondary thought processes to occur. The patient's usual type of response after the hypnotic session is to express amazement that such a trivial "sin" could have caused such long-enduring symptoms.

The traditional therapist is more apt to express skepticism than amazement. He will postulate that the specific trauma is not really the source of the trouble and that letting the patient believe it constitutes using an inexact interpretation to cover over the "true" dynamic issues. For now, I'll only point out that the material produced by the patients in this manner has strong emotional accompaniments which indicate it to be of some psychological significance; also, working with that material quickly produces profound changes that are long-enduring. Later, after describing the other techniques, I will discuss some thoughts on the correctness of the interpretations.

There is another objection which could be raised to this technique. Because the patient is able to respond only "yes" or "no," all the questions must be leading questions, and therefore it is possible to lead the patient to an answer preconceived by the therapist. This is more than likely if the "no's" are treated as resistances while the "yes's" are treated as confirmations (as occurred in the analysis of Little Hans). Here, though, the negative responses are given as much credence as the positive ones, so it is much less likely the patient will be led; his responses will be the compass bearings to lead the therapist.

There is another question of major importance which cannot be answered satisfactorily: "How does the therapist or the patient know the answers given by the fingers are the correct answers?" Undoubtedly, the patient could deliberately give false answers if he chose to do so. Patients can, and do, give false answers without hypnosis, and there is nothing about hypnosis which deprives them of that ability. Without deliberately choosing to falsify answers, the patient could still give incorrect ones, as happens also in traditional therapy.

The only real measure of the answers, other than attempting to obtain confirmation from outside sources, is the clinical improvement that follows, and even that is not altogether reliable, for the skeptic could be correct, and inexact interpretations may have done their job in an unusually effective manner. The changes which occur, however, are far-reaching and long-lasting and have come from data produced by the patient. The data may not conform to what analytic theory would have predicted, but rejecting data on that basis alone is not consistent with impartial observation.

Another question, for which the answer has at least partial confirmation, is, "Do the answers really come from the unconscious?" Patients consciously know the answers to some of the questions, but other questions and answers evoke comments like, "I didn't remember that at all until we did this work," or "I absolutely knew the answer would be 'yes,' so I was completely surprised when my finger answered 'no' instead." It is difficult to believe that answers which evoke such comments would have come only from conscious sources.

THE AFFECT BRIDGE

This technique, described by John Watkins (1971) [emanating from the work of Breuer and Freud (1955)], is a beautiful example of how hypnotic procedures can speed the recovery of repressed material and the affects associated to that material. In more traditional styles of therapy, the patient may associate an event in his present life to one in his earlier life, but most frequently the association is one of concepts or perceptions, with the emotional connection being absent, or at least unrecognized. If the emotional connection is not made, fascinating intellectual discussions may ensue but little change occurs.

Using the affect bridge, the patient is brought directly back to an original traumatic incident rather than arriving at it through the many steps of a long and circuitous free association. The connection between the past and the present is made by connecting feelings rather than by connecting mere ideas, and consequently the therapeutic gains accrue more quickly.

The technique itself is surprisingly simple. When an affect of unknown origin is present, either as a major difficulty in the patient's life or as an occurrence during the course of his therapy, he can be hypnotized and told to experience the affect again. He can be instructed to give some signal when he has the feeling ("Nod your head 'yes' when you have it") and then to let the feeling become more and more intense. Since the affect being investigated is usually an unpleasant one, prudence is in order as to how intense the therapist wishes it to become.

Next, the patient is told, "We will use the feeling as a bridge to the past. You will travel over that bridge to the very first time you ever experienced the feeling. As I count backward from ten to zero, you will travel backward to an earlier time, to another place. You will experience yourself getting smaller and smaller, younger and younger, until, at the count of zero, you will be reexperiencing the situation that first produced the feeling. Do not try to remember, do not try to do anything. Just let it happen and let yourself experience it." (It is an interesting observation that some patients do report feeling themselves getting smaller and younger as the therapist counts backward, while others do not have the same experience, suddenly finding themselves at the count of zero as being whatever size and age were appropriate to the situation being investigated.)

The therapist can usually discern from the patient's facial expressions and bodily postures that some event of significant emotional impact is taking place. The therapist asks the patient, "Describe what is happening now," or "How old are you now?" or "Where are you now?" etc. Depending on what the patient responds, the therapist asks further questions to help bring out what is taking place. In this manner an immediate emotional connection has been made between the affect manifest in the patient's current life and the origin of the affect, and valuable supplementary data can be obtained.

The patient does not always return to the original source of the affect; the age regression technique might not work at all or the patient "regresses" to some point at which the affect had been evoked but does not regress all the way back to the original time it came forth. Clinical judgment will usually assist the therapist in deciding if he has regressed to the origin of the symptom or has stopped at some station along the way. In the latter instance there can be a discussion of the material that was produced and then another journey undertaken to reach still further back into the patient's history.

Although it may be necessary to do some working-through procedures after using this technique, not infrequently it is found that the simple "reliving" of the original incident will suffice to relieve the patient of the unwanted feelings and to produce marked changes in his behavior.

The incidents uncovered are most commonly in the age range of eighteen months to six years, but incidents from earlier or much later in the patient's life are not infrequent. An example of an actual case might be helpful at this point.

The Case of John

John was a moderately successful 42-year-old businessman who sought treatment for a variety of symptoms he was having. His most distressing symptom was excessive use of cocaine; there were multiple dynamics involved with that particular symptom and helping him stop using it took several months. During the course of therapy another symptom became prominent: a crisis with a girlfriend brought him face to face with the realization that he really disliked women except for sexual activity—and yet didn't want to lose this one. He had no conscious knowledge of why he would dislike women except for a vague, "maybe it's because my mother treated me badly." Almost parenthetically he also mentioned he had been having stomach pains for as long as he could remember.

The affect bridge was explained to him and he was agreeable to trying it. We had used hypnosis previously; he was a good responder and went into a trance quickly. I suggested he let himself reexperience his feeling of disliking women and then let that feeling grow stronger and stronger. When that was accomplished we used age regression, and when I counted down to zero, his body suddenly contracted into an almost fetal position, his face contorted with apparent fear and pain, and he commenced crying, whimpering sounds.

He was asked to describe what was happening, and he said he was in bed and his stomach was hurting. A number of questions were needed to obtain much elaboration, but it turned out he was experiencing himself as a two-day-old infant in a hospital crib. His stomach was hurting from hunger. He had been crying, and "a woman in a white dress and white cap" picked him up, shook him roughly, then put him back into his crib, unfed. He continued whining and whimpering until I told him the incident was now over, he was returning to the year 1979 as a strong, mature adult, and now that he knew how he first developed a dislike for women, perhaps he could begin to feel differently.

There were no further working-through efforts made in the office, but the next week he told me that he was beginning to feel entirely differently about women and his stomach hadn't hurt him all week. We continued working on his other problems but did not address his feelings about women or his stomach problems again except for occasional inquiries as to how those symptoms were doing. They did not return during the next months of therapy, and when I saw him two years later for concerns about an eye injury he had suffered, neither symptom had returned.

This and similar cases are perplexing. The "reexperiencing" of events occurring after the age of three is not difficult to believe, but how do we explain such vivid recollections at day one or two of life? There are those who believe *all* our experiences are stored somewhere in our memory banks, and there should be no surprise in finding such memories recounted if the proper uncovering techniques are used. There is no firm evidence to support this belief; in fact, there are indications it is not true.

Loftus and Loftus (1980) raise serious questions about the validity of old memories evoked by electrode stimulation of the cerebral cortex, by hypnosis, or even by psychoanalysis. The user of each of those techniques is more likely to attest to the validity of the technique than objective evidence would warrant.

The traditional therapist will insist the patient's experience could be nothing more than a screen memory and any improvement the patient enjoys is the result of the screen memory shoring up his defenses against recognition of the true dynamics of his neurotic symptoms. If the latter explanation is correct and if the reliving of a screen memory plus the mild suggestion offered can so efficiently eliminate years of disturbing symptomatology, perhaps we should consider making more use of screen memories. Perhaps we do already, but if the screen memory fits into whatever theoretical framework we are using, and if that memory is consistent with our theory, then we don't recognize it as a screen. If the memory evoked by hypnosis is accurate, on the other hand, and there can be no way of knowing this, then some classical analytic theories may need to be reconsidered. There will be more said about that later.

As perplexing as the infantile memories may be, even more perplexing are the cases in which the affect bridge leads back to a "prior existence." This sounds so bizarre to most people that I would be hesitant to mention it, except for the fact therapists working with the affect bridge will occasionally uncover this response and should be prepared to handle it.

Although I do not believe in reincarnation and readily tell my patients so if the topic arises, I treat "prior life experiences" with respect. The manifest contents of dreams will often prove more bizarre than these experiences, but both seem to have important psychological significance and neither should be dismissed casually. These experiences, for reasons I cannot explain, almost always lead to rapid improvements in the patients' lives. Another case will serve as an example.

The Case of Shirley

Shirley is a legal secretary in her late thirties, married to an attorney; he accompanied her to each visit. She is intelligent and articulate and is doing well in her profession. Her husband stays home to take care of their two children, an arrangement they both enjoy. Shirley's complaint was her inability to fully enjoy sex, although she could find it mildly enjoyable if she had fantasies of being bound and raped. She associated intercourse with violence but had no conscious ideas as to why she had that association. Her fantasies caused me to suspect there was some fear of being "responsible" for her own sexual activity, hence the enjoyment only when bound and raped, but inquiries directed along those lines yielded no hints that fear of this responsibility was related to her problem.

A significant element in her personal history was her mother's development of tuberculosis when Shirley was only two years old. Her mother was sent to a TB sanitorium and never again displayed the closeness and affection she had once displayed (or Shirley imagined she had once displayed). Under hypnosis Shirley recalled a loving, almost erotic scene of being held in her mother's lap the night before the departure to the hospital and feelings of rage when her mother left. There were intense feelings of guilt because she had been so angry at her sick mother and the belief her mother had never again been affectionate because of that.

A tentative hypothesis was made: The loving scene with her mother, followed by the rage, may have started an association between sexual feelings and anger and/or violence. Further search along those lines did not produce what I considered supporting evidence for the hypothesis. I explained the affect bridge, and she agreed to try it.

Shirley described a scene in which she was a newborn infant and saw a woman, her mother, bleeding to death after her delivery. Since this was contrary to her known history, I asked what year it was, and she replied, "1793." In response to further questions, she said her family lived in a log cabin in the woods. Her father had been gone on a fur-trapping expedition, and a neighbor had acted as midwife, taking care of her after her mother's death. The session ended with our mutual surprise at the material produced.

She and her husband returned the next week, reporting sex had definitely improved for them, but now Shirley was aware of two other fears she associated to the sexual act: the fear she might harm someone else and the fear someone might harm her. Without hypnosis she could offer no information about either fear.

We used the affect bridge to examine her fear of harming someone else and she described a scene in a grand ballroom where she was attending a dance. She could not describe with certainty the year or other details, but it sounded as though it might be in nineteenth century France. Her husband was home, ill, and she became sexually involved with another man. Her husband learned of her infidelity, died shortly thereafter, and she blamed herself for his death.

The following week the couple reported their lovemaking had become even more enjoyable, and although Shirley no longer feared hurting someone else, she was still frightened of being hurt. The affect bridge was used again, and this time she described herself as a 15-year-old girl in fifteenth century Spain. She was painfully raped by her father, and he continued to have a painful (to her) incestuous relationship for some time after that.

At the next session she reported she was feeling free and happy during lovemaking and was enjoying it as she never had before. We terminated after a total of seven sessions. A number of months later her husband returned, seeking therapy to help him come to decisions regarding a return to an active role in his profession versus continuing with his present lifestyle. He reported the gains his wife had made were being maintained well, to their mutual delight.

It is easy to assume, as I did, that the maternal mortality in the log cabin and the incestuous relationship in Spain were both screen memories. The maternal mortality in the log cabin could be, perhaps, a screen for Shirley's wish to kill her mother for the desertion occurring when she was a young girl, or a screen for a fear she had caused her mother's illness in real life instead of in the log cabin, or for the wish to be rid of her mother in order to have her father to herself. The scene in Spain could be a screen for real or fantasized incestuous relations with her own father in the twentieth century.

I did not pursue the possibilities mentioned above arising from the scene in the log cabin, but I did attempt to look more closely at the incidents in the Spanish scene. I explained I believed her Spanish drama could be a cover for events that had occurred or had been fantasized in this life, and perhaps it was easier for her to speak of a young girl in Spain than to speak of herself and more current events. She agreed to return to my office a few months later so we could use hypnosis to explore that possibility. That exploration yielded no new information.

She told me she had been willing to try to find new data but she had had serious questions about the validity of my hypothesis. She had spent two years in analysis in another community because of her sexual problems, and incest fantasies had been the major focus of that analysis. The fantasies had seemed so real to her that she had written her parents to see if some of the things had actually happened, much to her parents' distress. She declared, "If I was able to talk with my analyst then about myself and my fantasies, I shouldn't have to avoid talking about myself with you."

I do not accept reincarnation explanations for this case and would be much more inclined to accept screen memories as an explanation. That being true, I cannot argue against the screen memory theory for data retrieved from "in utero" scenes or from scenes said to have occurred in the first days of life. It is entirely conceivable to me, however, that neither explanation is necessarily true, and some theory, as yet unannounced, may lead to a better understanding. For instance, the patient was instructed to "return to the first time you ever experienced this feeling," and it is possible the first time was in a childhood dream.

Adults have dreams which leave them with strong feelings of fear, sorrow, etc., for hours or even days after they awaken. It is not unreasonable to believe children have similar dreams, but the affect is so overwhelming that regression begins almost immediately, and later, in adult life, conventional uncovering techniques do not remove the repression. If a major portion of Shirley's analysis had dealt with incestuous fantasies from childhood, it is almost certain she would have had dreams about incest as a child. Daytime residues arising from adventure or romantic stories could have shaped the manifest content of the dreams, and when (if) hypnosis lifted the repression, the reexperiencing of the dream would appear to be experiencing events from a former life. This speculation is not offered as explanation, only as an example of a possible alternative.

If such an explanation were true, and here I am not merely playing around with words, the events from the "prior life" would not be a screen memory for incestuous wishes. They would be the recollection of an actual traumatic experience, a dream.

If the screen memory theory is true, however, and a few sessions of this technique provided more improvement in the patient's life than two years of a traditional analysis, then we should carefully reconsider our objections to screen memories. It would not suffice to believe screen memories obscure the "real" dynamics and therefore no significant change could occur and be maintained. Significant changes do occur and are maintained.

ourse, the case illustrations presented do not prove the validity of this technique. The symptom ablation occurring is not comparable to the benefits of a full analysis. There are no before and
after objective measurements to confirm that improvement had
occurred at all. All there is in the way of evidence are the declara-
tions made by the patients, and by the husband of one, that their
lives were better and they had found the therapy had accomplished
what they were seeking. This evidence should not be discarded
lightly, however, by those who do not have more convincing evidence to justify the validity of their own techniques.

EGO STATE THERAPY

John and Helen Watkins, both at the University of Montana,
were the first to describe this remarkable uncovering technique.
In large measure their work is somewhat similar to Gestalt and
transactional analysis techniques, but theoretically it is based upon
the writings of Federn (1952), who first described ego states. Un-
fortunately, Federn's descriptions make for exceedingly difficult
reading, and that, perhaps, has accounted for his relative anonymity.
According to the Watkins (1979), an ego state "consists of those
behaviors, perceptions and experiences which are bound together
by some common principles and separated by a boundary from other
such states."

The Watkins (1979) postulate that regression, via hypnosis or
more traditional therapies, reactivates the ego state of the age to
which the patient regresses. Information and feelings contained
within the ego state then become accessible to study and, consequently, to alteration. Although the ego state represents only one
facet of the patient's personality, it appears to be much like a
separate personality dwelling within the patient.

In effect, it is almost as though each of us were a multiple personality, but with one major difference. In the true multiple personality, the boundaries between the ego states are so impermeable
that the actions of one ego state may occur without another ego
state being aware of those actions. Thus, the person may have a

wild, debauched night out on the town with no recollection of it the next day when another ego state is predominant. In those of us not afflicted, or blessed, with this malady, the different ego states may cause us to act in ways we do not understand, but at least we are aware of our actions. The illustration I offer to patients, which they immediately understand, is, "Damn, a part of me wants to do this, but another part just won't let me!"

Using hypnosis, the therapist can speak directly to these parts, and they can speak back. They can reveal when they first came into existence, what caused their formation, and what they are attempting to accomplish. What they are attempting to accomplish is almost always a laudable goal, but their methods may leave much to be desired. Their goals must often be reformulated by the therapist into a more positive concept. For example, if the part is punishing the patient for being bad, this can be redefined as trying to make the patient a better person. If the part is causing repeated failures, this may be redefined as protecting the patient from the imagined or real dangers of success; the redefinitions, however, can be made successfully only if they are congruent with other data given by the part. *Positive redefining of the part's goal is an important step in this technique and greatly enhances its effectiveness.*

At times the parts are almost classic examples of an id, an ego, or a superego, although they may arise at ages not generally thought to be productive of those Freudian constructs. The parts may be classic examples of Berne's (1964) Parent, Child, or Adult. At times the parts do not seem to fit those concepts at all. Some of the parts may appear to be pure defensive mechanisms. It is impossible to know in advance how many parts will appear, but generally it will be found there is at least one part involved in each symptomatic behavior, and the part involved in that behavior may be in great conflict with another part striving for an opposite behavior. In my experience, therapy falters or fails when many more than five or six parts make their appearances, but to hear from so many different portions of the patient's psyche is relatively uncommon.

The number of ego states elicited depends in part on how many different, unrelated symptoms are being treated, and in part on the manner in which the therapist is doing his job. It is conceivable a therapist could call forth a part who causes excessive drinking, a part who causes reckless driving, and another part who causes sexual promiscuity—or the therapist could call forth one part who causes self-destructive behavior. When possible, it is better to seek the one part rather than the three.

Frequently, the parts can be dealt with individually, one after the other, depending upon the problems the patient presents. At other times, however, the parts are in such conflict with one another, or so untrusting of one another, that it becomes necessary to do "group therapy" with the one individual patient. In one patient, for example, the "Punisher," a superego-like element, would not stop causing panic attacks because he did not trust the "Adventurer" to desist from certain activities the Punisher considered immoral. The Adventurer, a beautiful example of the id, would not desist because he feared the Punisher would never let the patient have fun again. As a result of carefully negotiated compromises and use of "Stability," the ego element, as arbitrator, the panic attacks subsided, the patient found new enjoyment in socially acceptable activities and became able, once again, to live a happy, productive life. The overall changes were profound: not only was the specific target symptom—panic attacks—relieved, but he no longer found it necessary to be excessively competitive in a number of different areas of his life, and an obsessive approach to work and social activity gave way to a more relaxed style of living and more time devoted to his wife and family. Data derived from this patient indicate the obsessive behavior, all in highly commendable fields of endeavor, had been to defend against feelings of shame derived from childhood activity.

The names used in this brief case description are another interesting aspect of this technique. Almost every part has a name and will tell its name when asked. The names are often a surprise to the patient, particularly when they are common, given names, like Sam or Mary. The patient frequently has no idea where the name came from; at other times the patient may suddenly recall, "I remember now; when I was . . . . . . (the age at which the ego state appeared),

I had a friend named Sam who ......" (something similar to what the patient had been doing or feeling). The descriptive names, like those in the case above, are much easier to understand.

In addition to having names, the parts usually have ages and genders. The ages are consonant with the age at which the part appeared; also, when that part is speaking, the speech patterns and body language are often, but not always, congruent. The gender of the part often appears based upon stereotyped concepts of what masculine or feminine behavior should be. Almost all the female patients with whom I have worked displayed at least one male part; female parts in male patients appear less often during the course of therapy.

When doing ego state therapy, these are the steps I follow. There is no need for the reader to memorize the steps, for once the principle is understood, they flow naturally, one after the other. Other therapists undoubtedly modify the procedure to better fit their own styles.

1) Explain the concept to the patient before inducing the hypnotic state. I've done the therapy without first explaining it to the patient and it works just as well, but some patients feel frightened of having "multiple personalities" unless the explanation is given in advance.

2) After the hypnotic induction, ask to speak with the part that is causing some specific behavior or feeling. "I wish to speak with that part that causes you to. . . . When that part is there, please say, 'I am here.' "

3) When the part announces its presence, thank it for appearing and ask, "What is your name, part?" (It may also be asked its gender, if that is not apparent from the name.)

4) Ask how old the whole person was when the part first appeared. Encourage dissociation by proper use of pronouns: "How old was *she* when *you* first appeared?" Note: The ego state is usually "young," so I prefer to address it in simple language.

5) Ask what was happening to the whole person that caused the part to appear and perhaps obtain elaboration on those events.

6) If possible, try to define what the goal of the part was: "So you were there to help her (punish her, comfort her, etc.), is that right?"

7) Comment on the value of the goal, redefined in positive terms.

8) Offer a better method for obtaining those goals and ask the part's cooperation in trying those new methods. If the part is reluctant, suggest trying the new methods for only one week to see how they work out.

9) Thank the part for its information and cooperation and assure it you will check with it next visit to see how things are going. Then tell it, "You may go back where you came from."

10) Awaken the patient with, "When I count backward from three, the whole person will awaken and will remember all of this that can be handled comfortably."

In order to best demonstrate this technique and to show what the results of it can be, two more case presentations will be used. The first case will include a verbatim transcript of the first session of ego state therapy. It will show how the technique is explained to the patient and how the therapist then goes about using it.

The Case of Jennifer

Jennifer is a 28-year-old single woman, attractive, intelligent and with a good sense of humor. She was working part-time and going to school part-time to become a professional in a medically allied field. She sought therapy "to learn why I engage in so much self-destructive behavior."

In our first session, conducted without hypnosis, she told me she abused alcohol and amphetamines, had had sixteen automobile accidents, and had entered one destructive relationship after another. One of her lovers had committed suicide two years ago, and another had attempted suicide three days before she came to this appointment. Her fantasies and dreams were almost all of brutal self-mutilation.

Both parents were alcoholic. She was raised primarily by her father and had been "the boy" he wanted. She maintained a basically masculine role until entering junior high school, when she "became a girl all of a sudden," and became totally immersed in her new, exciting girlish role. Her sense of humor enabled her to be the class clown, in the best sense of that word; her friendliness allowed her to enjoy a large circle of friends; and her intelligence permitted her to make excellent grades. She was the most stable member of her family and was thrust into the role of becoming the family counselor.

When she graduated to high school, there was another sudden and marked change in her identity. She went from a very straight life to a hippie lifestyle. She moved to the Haight-Ashbury section of San Francisco and immersed herself in that subculture of the sixties. For reasons she could not explain, she left that scene and joined a strict fundamentalist religion. She left the religion when she and another member of the church formed a lesbian relationship. It was that friend who had committed suicide two years previously.

Her second session was spent mostly in telling me of her current relationship with the lover who had recently attempted suicide. She explained she felt trapped into staying with that lover for fear of another suicide attempt. Her lover had specifically threatened suicide if she did leave. I spoke briefly of the dangers of letting herself be blackmailed by such threats and then told her I often use hypnosis with my patients and thought it might be useful for her.

She was agreeable to the idea, and I sensed she even relished it as though it were another dangerous adventure on which she could embark. She proved to be an excellent subject, and after being hypnotized, awakened, and rehypnotized, she was told we would start the actual work on her next visit. A transcript of that visit follows.

Permission is requested for recording the session, and Jennifer agrees.

T. There seems to be a part of you that's self-destructive; another part wants to go ahead and function well. Part of you knows it's not good to drink, that you shouldn't get involved in these destructive relationships, and yet a part of you seems to drive you into that anyway. The psychological body has parts just as the physical body does. Most people can relate to that immediately—"part of me wants to do this, and another part just won't let me."

Now, under hypnosis we can speak with those parts. It's an intriguing process. The parts will usually have names. They might be regular names, like Betty, Sue, or Jack, or descriptive names like Fear, Anger, or whatever. They will also have sexes. Almost every female patient I have worked with has had at least one male-gendered part; I don't see the female parts in the male patients as often, but they are there.

Each of these parts generally has its own age, having been "born" during some traumatic episode in the patient's life. Almost always these parts are trying to help you in one way or another, even the self-destructive ones. They might be trying to punish you for past "sins" to make you a better person; they might be doing other things. It's as if these parts learned one way of doing things at the moment they were born and then were sealed off and have not been able to accept new data. Under hypnosis it's as if we open up the capsule and are able to give them new information so they can achieve whatever their goals are, but are able to achieve them in ways that are more productive than what they used to do.

I do not try to get rid of parts. They're very strong; they are very powerful; they are a part of you. I admire and appreciate that strength and intend to have you take advantage of it. By talking to these parts, we can find other ways for them to behave and let them achieve their goals in a more successful manner. All right, that's what I would like to do today—to talk to that part that has been causing self-destructive behavior, to learn why it came into your life, what it's trying to accomplish, and see if it can accomplish that in a more useful manner. Are there any questions about that?

P. Yeah, I do have one question. How could that one part of me that's self-destructive be of any use to me at all? I mean, you maintain you don't want to get rid of it?

T. Well, let's say, for instance, it's doing all these things to punish you. What it's really trying to do, then, is make you a better person, and what I would try to do is enlist its aid to help you become a better person in other ways; for instance, like a conscience to warn you, "No, don't do that, that's bad," or to punish you mildly if you do something bad, so you're less likely to do it again. And to give you a pat on the back when you've done something good, and in a sense push you to do good things to make up for whatever bad things you might have done in the past. So it could be very strong and useful for you in those ways.

I don't know what it's doing or why it's doing it, so those are just guesses or examples of how it sometimes works out. Any other questions?

P. Nope.

T. Okay, let's go on with it then. We'll start kind of like we did the first time. One . . . roll your eyeballs to the very top of your head; feel the strain. Two . . . slowly close your eyelids and take a deep breath. Good. Three . . . let the breath out. Let the eye muscles relax. Let yourself just float back into the hypnotic state. Let it flow all through you, taking over more and more. Relaxing your body, relaxing your brain, going more and more deeply, more and more comfortably into the hypnotic state so we can use this state to understand and change what has been going on in your life.

I am going to count backward from ten, and with each number you can let yourself go further into the hypnotic state, so by the time I get to zero, you will have gone so deeply I can speak with the different parts of your personality and they can speak with me. Ten, nine, eight, deeper and deeper. Seven, six, five, four, just letting yourself go further and further into it. Three, two, one, zero. Deep, deep, deep.

There is a part of you that has been driving you to self-destruction by use of alcohol and other drugs, by automobile accidents, by bad, harmful relationships—and I imagine that part has been doing this for reasons that seem good to it. I would like to get to know and understand that part. When that part is there, I would like to speak to it. I want that part to come forward so I can speak with it. When it is there, I want it to say, "I am here."

P. I am here.

T. Thank you for coming out, Part. Do you have a name I can call you?

P. Bad.

T. Bad? All right, are you a male or a female part?

P. Female.

T. All right, thank you. And how old was the whole person when you first appeared?

P. Three.

T. So you've been with her a long time, is that right? What was happening that caused you to come into her life?

P. (long pause) Competition.

T. Competition? Competition with whom?

P. My older sister. (Note the response is "My older sister," not, "Her older sister," indicating less depersonalization than I would like to see. My questions will continue to emphasize the separation between the part and the whole person, and the patient's responses will change.)

T. *She* was competing with *her* older sister then? How was she competing?

P. Trying to get attention from her parents. (The part is now using the third person to describe the patient.)

T. And how did she try to get attention from her parents?

P. She'd do anything to get attention.

T. And did you feel sorry for her because she wasn't getting enough attention?

P. Yes.

T. So you were there to help her get attention? (Beginning to define a positive aspect of the part's activity.)

P. Uh-hunh.

T. And is that what you've been trying to do ever since, help her get attention?

P. Uh-hunh.

T. So it sounds as if you're a friend of hers, trying to help her get attention. Is that right?

P. Uh-hunh.

T. And certainly when she gets in an automobile accident, that brings a lot of attention, doesn't it? And I guess when she drinks too much, or uses drugs of other sorts, that gets a lot of attention too, doesn't it?

P. Uh-hunh.

T. So you've really been trying to help her, by letting her get attention by doing these things. Was it your feeling she could not get attention by doing good things?

P. (pause, sigh) Sometimes it doesn't work. It doesn't work to be good to get attention. Some days you just get used.

T. That's true. Sometimes it does work, though, doesn't it?

P. Uh-hunh.

T. Tell me, does it always work to do bad things?

P. No, there's a certain satisfaction in getting away with things, though. But no, it doesn't always work. Sometimes it hurts.

T. How do you feel when it hurts her?

P. Sad.

T. Do you think she's capable of getting attention by doing good things, by using her intelligence, maturity, judgment, and energy? Is she capable of getting attention just by doing good things?

P. Somehow it goes against her grain.

T. Sure. Well, you've been doing things one way for a long, long time, and it's often difficult doing things in another way, isn't it? (Acknowledging the hesitancy to change, which we often see in patients with any form of therapy.)

P. Uh-hunh.

T. But since you're her friend, since you want her to get attention, and since it makes you feel bad when things turn out to hurt her, could you consider the possibility of doing things a different way?

P. Uh-hunh.

T. I believe what you'll find is that she's a very bright person, with lots of energy. She's capable of good judgment, and she's capable of getting a lot of good attention by doing good things in her life. At school or on a job, she can get much better attention from healthy, stable people she'll get into a relationship with than she could with the losers she connects up with. She certainly gets a lot of attention from those losers, but it brings her down, it's painful to her, and it makes her feel trapped in those relationships. (Using information the patient had told me in our first session, and therefore it is all reasonable to her.)

P. Yeah.

T. And if she were with winners rather than losers, in some ways she might not get as much attention, but the kind of attention would be so much better it would make up for that. Can you see that?

P. Uh-hunh. I want to say, lately I've been dying.

T. What's killing you?

P. Jennifer's more in touch with the poor choices she makes in relationships, and I've really stifled her and it's not fun anymore to be bad. I'm stuck and I feel stuck.

T. Well, look, I don't want you to die. You're her friend. You've been with her a long time, and you give her strength and energy. You've been forcing her to do all kinds of things, even though in a sense she didn't want to do them. If a part of her has that much strength and energy, I think it's a very important part of her, but I'd like you to start using that power you have in new directions. I think it's splendid you want her to get attention, but the quality of the attention needs to be changed. And I think competition is healthy if there are are reasonable limits. You can come to her aid when she feels it's important to compete, but when it's important to compete in healthier ways, not to do just anything to get attention, but to get good, healthy attention by good, healthy behavior. Change your direction to help her with that, and you can be a very wonderful friend of hers and a very important part of her life. You'll be a welcome ally for her. And I don't believe she would want to kill you or have you die, if you changed your direction of behavior. Does that sound appealing to you?

P. Umm, it sounds wonderful.

T. Okay, now look, you've been doing things one way for a long, long time. I don't anticipate you'll be able to change all of that overnight, but with just a little bit of practice and experience, you'll find things moving in the right direction again. She, and certainly I, will be patient while you're going through this learning period. You might make some mistakes, but we'll be looking for improvement, not perfection.

P. Uh, you know, she's afraid of being bored. I come out a lot of times and it gets to be self-destructive. She's afraid she's not gonna get enough. She's not gonna have a good enough time, she's not gonna be noticed enough, she's not gonna do well enough, so she goes to extremes and that's when it turns into hurting.

T. Do you know if there's another part that might cause her to feel that way?

P. (long silence)

T. Maybe you don't. Maybe you haven't met such a part, I don't know. Look, you seem to have a lot of creativity. You've certainly created a lot of bad situations that have caused trouble, so I'd like you to start using your creativity to create good situations that get attention for her. As I said, it may take a little while for you to be able to get this under control, but I believe you'll find you can do it much more quickly than you imagine you can. I think you'll find the results are very, very pleasing. You'll find there are healthy activities that are just as much fun as unhealthy or dangerous ones; there are safe activities that can be just as much fun as unsafe ones. So I want you to start using your power and your creativity in these ways.

P. Okay.

T. Well, Bad, I kind of hate to keep calling you Bad because I think you've been trying to be helpful, but just in the wrong directions. I'll just keep calling you Bad until you come up with another name for me to call you.

P. Uh-hunh. I don't really like the name either.

T. Okay. I think you've been very cooperative, and I truly appreciate the information you have given me. I appreciate your willingness to try to change things. Do you have any questions or comments you'd like to ask of me?

P. Uh, maybe I've been putting thoughts into Jennifer's mind to take things that aren't hers, and she's guilty about the fact she's been taking more than she deserves. Money from her parents. Selfish thoughts, taking things.

T. Has she actually taken things?

P. Yes.

T. And did you get her to take those things because she was feeling deprived?

P. Uh-hunh.

T. In what ways was she feeling deprived?

P. Ohhh, she's been psychologically beaten so she deserves to borrow money with no intention of paying it back, or going out and blowing it on drugs, or going out to dinner. Things like that. I just tell her she's paid her dues, and she has to override her guilt after she does it, and she turns around and fools herself and tries to fool her conscience, gets drugs, and screws up, and it turns into a vicious cycle.

T. Well, it may be true in many ways she was psychologically beaten down, but you can see that getting her to do this causes guilt feelings that beat her down even more. She doesn't end up feeling better because of this; she ends up feeling worse, doesn't she?

P. Uh-hunh.

T. But again, I would say you've been trying to be her friend. You've had the idea if she stole these things it would repay her and it would make her feel better. I would say I think your motives have been splendid, but your methods of operating haven't been working, so we have to find new ways of operating that will make her feel better instead of making her feel worse.

P. Yeah. But it's so familiar. It's such a long-standing way of dealing with her. It's so familiar. It's so easy for her to listen, to obey that. (Again, hesitancy to change.)

T. Okay, it's you she's listening to, and it's you who have to start making the corrections. You've been her friend, you've been trying to make her feel better, but you know making her do this kind of thing makes her feel worse. You'll have to start putting other ideas into her head, more constructive ideas. Tell me, how do you think her parents would react if she started becoming more the "good girl" they wanted her to be?

P. They would be very pleased.

T. And she'd probably get a great deal of attention from that, wouldn't she? And I imagine they'd be very happy to lend her money or to give her money if they knew she could behave in socially acceptable, constructive ways. Do you think they'd be willing to do that?

P. Uh-hunh. For a while behaving badly and getting the kind of attention she got was nurturing; she would get nurturing, a real intense concern, but now it's just a rejection when she behaves that way, so it's not as intense a concern. The intensity isn't there, but it's much more satisfying.

T. So, if she starts "behaving," you think she will start getting a lot of attention again, and of a much better quality, is that right?

P. Uh-hunh.

T. Okay, I think you see what your task is, and as I said, there's no need for you to die. I hope you don't, because with your power, if you start working in this new direction, you can get her a great deal of attention of a very fine quality. Do you have any other comments or any other questions?

P. I feel a lot better about being a part of her.

T. Sure, and you'll become a very valuable part of her and she's going to feel a lot better. Rather than having another part fighting against you all the time, she'll accept you as a real ally, and you and the other part will be working in the same direction. Rather than wasting energy fighting against one

another, you'll find you'll be using your energies working toward the same goals. She'll feel stronger, more healthy, a lot
more put together.

P. Uh, you know, I feel a real apology toward her.

T. I don't know if that's even necessary, because you were trying to
help her, and you certainly owe her no apology for that. You
got stuck at a very early age into thinking you could help her
in one particular way. If you still behave that same way now
you'll owe her an apology, now that you see the difference.
Right now, she owes you a debt of gratitude for being her
friend and for working so hard in her behalf. There will be a
great deal of relief now that you can work in other directions,
but nonetheless you have been a good and faithful friend of
hers. She'll learn to love and appreciate you when she sees
you've learned to work in these new directions.

P. I'll buy that!

T. Thank you for your information and your cooperation, and I'd
like to talk with you again next week to see how things are
going, to see what other changes or corrections we might want
to make, and to see if there are other parts we might want to
speak with. So you can go back to where you come from, with
great relief. There's no need for you to die for Jennifer to work
her life out better; as a matter of fact, your being there will be
of great help to her.

 Now, I'll count backward from three, and the whole person
will awaken. Three . . . two . . . one . . . zero. (Jennifer
awakens, looks around for a few moments to reorient herself.)
That was very interesting, wasn't it?

P. Ohh, it was! It felt like I was . . . I think it came out from way
down inside, like it had isolated itself, like you had it do, and I
was just next to it. (Laughs happily.)

T. Now I think you see what I mean about how these parts can be
useful to you?

P. Yeah! It's really interesting, because I took what came. I was real
relaxed. I just took whatever came, and what came surprised

me. It was like I was over here reacting to it. I feel so good about this session. I feel like something's been accomplished.

T. Certainly some understanding has been accomplished, and that's an important first step. The changes in behavior will determine how useful this accomplishment has been. Frequently the changes occur rather rapidly. There may be some fallings back to the old ways of doing things simply because bad habits of long standing are hard to break. You may find some real changes occurring this week.

P. There's a real relief knowing that part of me doesn't have to die, for when it has to die, it feels it has to act out in the extreme ways. As long as it feels it can be a part of me, it can work for me instead of against me. There's a hell of a lot of energy in it. (Laughs happily.) It's a real kicker, I'll tell you! I like it, it's fun! There's a real sense of humor in that aspect of me. (Tape runs out, and so does the session a minute or two later.)

Fourth Session (the second time we use ego state therapy): Jennifer comes into the session looking very bright and happy. She reports she is feeling much better. She decided to break off the relationship with her lover, and although she felt very bad about it for one day, she did not cruise the bars and get drunk the way she would have in the past. I congratulate her on the change. She says she has dropped the tough façade she had been using, is acting more open and friendly toward others, and is getting gratifying responses from them. She has the feling she is now her "real self."

She reports, however, there are times she suddenly starts crying for no known reason, and this has become a source of concern to her. I hypnotize her and ask for the part causing the crying; "Melancholy" responds. Melancholy says she appeared when Jennifer was five years old and her parents' drunken brawls were causing much anguish; she was there to provide release of Jennifer's feelings but had been repressed and was able to break through only on rare occasions, mostly when the feelings were inappropriate to what was going on. I reassure Melancholy her function is a valuable one, but much of the value is lost and troubles are caused when she forces out the feelings at inappropriate times. Melancholy agrees to stop coming out inappropriately if Jennifer will let her come out when it is appropriate. Jennifer agrees. (No further episodes of inappropriate crying occurred.)

Fifth Session: Jennifer reports this has been a bad week, with a relapse to the use of cocaine and the abuse of alcohol. Under hypnosis the part causing the relapse is identified as "Tough." Tough came into Jennifer's life when she was four to help her handle the problems in her family—"She was too young to go through that by herself." This part feels Jennifer will be weak and vulnerable without help to make her tough. I congratulate the part for helping Jennifer endure the many difficulties of her earlier life but point out there is a difference between toughness and strength, and now Tough can be of more use by helping Jennifer be strong without the tough façade. The part understands and agrees to change its mode of helping Jennifer. (There have been no further reported uses of cocaine, and the only reported use of excess alcohol was in happy celebration with some friends.)

Near the end of this session Jennifer says she has been seeing things in her life much more clearly since we started using the hypnosis, but she feels frightened of the clarity. She cannot explain the fear, and there is not enough time remaining in the session to explore it further.

Sixth Session: Jennifer has been overloading herself with constructive activities in school, on the job, and in helping friends. She is feeling really good about herself for the first time since junior high, and again refers to having much more "clarity," but being apprehensive of it. We use hypnosis and learn a part named "Kid" is afraid of the clarity because clarity means growing up and if Jennifer grows up, Kid is afraid there will be no place for her in Jennifer's life.

I express appreciation for the fun and joy Kid has brought to Jennifer and point out there will always be a place for this part in her life. As she grows up, though, there will be times and places for play and times and places for more serious endeavors. I suggest if Kid confines her activities to the appropriate times and places, she will be well appreciated and will always be a valuable, welcome part. Kid understands, no longer feels frightened, and agrees to cooperate. (The fears of clarity made no further appearance.)

Seventh and Eighth Sessions: We do not use hypnosis. Jennifer spends the time primarily reporting on what is going on in her life. She is doing very well at work and has received a promotion. She enjoys her newfound feelings of closeness to others. She's no longer harshly critical of herself. She's enjoying and amazed at the clarity with which she sees her world, and in the past few weeks has begun to relish learning things at school, going from C grades to A's. She sees this as a turning point in her life and believes it is now important to decide if she wants to continue her life as a lesbian or become heterosexual, seeing major problems with either decision.

Ninth Session: We use hypnosis to hear from the part that wants to remain gay. This part, named Lesbian, came into her life when she was five and reveals several dynamics involved. Her father wanted a son and treated her like one in many ways; this was accentuated when his only son was found to have birth defects and it was apparent he could never have a normal son. Lesbian was there to help win the father's approval.

Jennifer's mother was either physically or emotionally absent, and Jennifer had a longing, almost sexual in nature, for the love and affection of a woman. Being gay helped fulfill this longing. Jennifer really needed "nurturing" from any source and did not believe she could ever receive it from a man.

Jennifer developed a great hatred toward her father, and remaining a lesbian was one way to get revenge on him. She speaks with great intensity, actual revulsion, about her father.

Tenth Session: Jennifer reports a "fabulous" week. She's had a feeling of high self-esteem, feels more attractive, and is strongly motivated to make her life work out well. It has become clear to her that she must move out of the family's home in order to decide on the libidinal direction of her lifestyle and is making plans to make the move in the next few weeks. The great rage she had felt toward her father has markedly diminished and she feels empathy instead. (I had made no interventions in this regard.) She has become the family counselor again, enjoys that role much more than being the big burden on the family, and "I'm pleased as punch with myself."

We use hypnosis to speak with the part that wants her to become heterosexual. This part is "Jenny." Jenny came in junior high, at the time Jennifer had reported going from her tomboy image to becoming a girl all of a sudden. Jenny believed a gay life would be less fulfilling than a heterosexual one and thought Jennifer was selling herself short believing she could never receive nurturing from a man. Men really loved Jennifer, but they always approached her as "good old funny, reliable Jennifer, one of the boys" or as an object for "raw sex."

Jenny says Jennifer is actually beginning to act more feminine, and during the last quarter of school was aided by one of her professors who treated her like a woman and who offered much nurturing in an adult way. Jennifer felt she was falling in love with the professor and thoroughly enjoyed the experience.

I ask Lesbian to come out, and she does. She has heard the conversation with Jenny and agrees the two of them can work together to help Jennifer. They both want her to be happy, to receive and give affection, to enjoy sex with someone she cares about, etc. They will see what they can do in a cooperative fashion to help her achieve these goals.

Eleventh Session: Jennifer is delighted with the way her life is going now. She enumerates the many improvements that have occurred and tells me she is currently "asexual." This does not bother her, for she feels it is a temporary period of growth during which she is learning to relate better to men and women as whole people rather than as sexual partners. She is growing to appreciate her male and female friends more, and they seem to reciprocate her feelings. She wishes to give herself time to develop relationships further and to sort out her desires to be homosexual, heterosexual, or bisexual. She is ready to terminate therapy at this time and will feel very comfortable about returning if she finds a need for further help in the future. She expresses her thanks; I express my pleasure at her successful use of the time spent; we terminate.

The Case of Robert

Robert, a displaced Texan and former paratrooper, was first seen in a crisis situation. Initially he would not even speak to me except to ask for paper and pen to write out what he was feeling. He furiously wrote of his wishes to destroy women in frighteningly primitive and brutal fashion. At 38 he was an exceedingly powerful-looking man, five foot ten, 275 pounds, with few of those pounds having gone to fat.

The intensity of his emotion was diminished by his writing, and he then calmly told me he was afraid he would lose control of his anger and hurt someone. On one occasion he had thrown his wife across a room, and on another he had taken a gun to find his brother-in-law and shoot him. On the latter occasion he had recognized the irrationality of his intent, had driven to a police station instead, and had given his gun to the police.

His life seemed to him to be one of endless frustration. His father had always belittled and berated him and had never been satisfied with any of his accomplishments. His father had died shortly before Robert had obtained a job of which his father might have been proud. He and his wife worked for his brother-in-law, and he felt belittled and unappreciated there, too. He had aspirations of going into business for himself but had neither the financial capabilities nor the confidence to do so. His children were sources of repeated aggravation.

He did not feel he could contain his frustrations much longer and felt desperate need for help. Because we were both concerned about his potential for violence, I referred him to a therapist in a hospital in a nearby community, and the patient and I were both relieved when he arrived there.

After a brief but intense stay in the hospital, he came out markedly changed. He had learned to recognize that much of his frustration had arisen from his failure to act appropriately in his own behalf and had gained a sense of being able to control himself and his life without needing to resort to violence.

The first two sessions after his hospitalization were spent in marital therapy, helping him and his wife recognize how some of his grievances had arisen, and helping him find better ways of dealing with the troublesome issues. They worked hard between visits, and by the third session they seemed to have corrected the issues that had threatened to lead to a dissolution of their marriage; they also were talking more openly and more intimately than they had ever done before. His main complaint then became his tendency to "freeze up" during certain sexual intimacies. He expressed concern that this symptom might have something to do with his childhood relationship to his mother when his father was gone for long periods of time but could not elaborate or even tell me why he thought this might be the source of trouble. He was amenable to the idea of using hypnosis to explore the issue and proved to be a good subject.

In the following session we started ego state therapy. When I asked to speak with the part which was afraid of intimacy, "Monster" came out. This part had developed when the patient was six and he and his family moved from the town in which they had been living. In the move he was forced to leave behind all his friends, his pet dog, and his pet cat. Those losses were so exceptionally painful to him that the Monster came to protect him from enduring similar losses in the future. Monster believed this could be done best by preventing him from becoming too intimate with anyone in the future. (Robert later wrote me a long account of his many childhood and adolescent frustrations arising from bungled attempts at sexual intimacy with seemingly available and willing women.)

I spoke with Monster and explained that his attempts to prevent Robert from being hurt again were certainly praiseworthy in their intent, but at this time in his adult life there was much less chance of his being hurt in the same ways as before, and protecting Robert from intimacy was also prohibiting him from having many of the pleasures life could offer. Besides, intimate relations with friends and family could provide a new source of protection, for then he would have caring people to comfort him if losses did occur. I added that we all need protection from becoming involved with people who are likely to cause us hurt, and Monster could serve an important function in offering this protection once he learned to distinguish the good guys from the bad. Monster understood what I was telling him, and although he felt a little frightened to change his tactics, he was willing to give it a try. He also said he would rather not be called Monster anymore but would prefer to be called "Friend."

At the following session, Robert expressed amazement and gratitude for the "remarkable improvement" which had occurred, and his wife, who had continued accompanying him to all the sessions, happily confirmed the improvement. We continued for a few more sessions working on other issues with ego state therapy; other parts involved in those other issues appeared, and improvements in those areas occurred almost as quickly. The improvements were not only maintained but became more manifest in broader spheres of his life during the ensuing two months as we worked less dramatically and less successfully in family therapy designed to improve relations between the parents and the children of the family.

Discussion

Here, again, we are faced with the question as to the real source of a symptom. Robert offered a possible clue to the source: his concern that it had something to do with his relationship to his mother while his father was gone on long business trips. There could not have been a more open invitation to the exploration of Oedipal issues, and if they had been pursued, undoubtedly they would have been found. If they had been worked with sufficiently, it is probable his symptom would have vanished as completely as it did using this other technique. But here we come to a question of paramount importance: If Oedipal issues had been found, and if working with those issues had ended his symptoms, would that necessarily mean they were the real source of his trouble? I offer the heretical proposition it need not.

Although concern is frequently expressed that hypnosis produces change by nothing more substantial than the process of suggestion, it could be true that traditional therapy produces change by nothing more substantial than the process of suggestion—and at a far slower rate. There has already been an exposition of my belief that a therapist can lead a patient to some predetermined goal (memory, thought, feeling). There is support for the possibility that the therapist can suggest a memory, and later the patient reports that memory as being his own (Dewald, 1972; Wolpe and Rachman, 1960; Loftus and Loftus, 1980). It is also possible that if the therapist were to make interpretations repeatedly which all imply, "The reason you freeze up when you have sexual intimacy with your wife is because you associate this to your wish to have sexual intimacy with your mother," the patient would begin to believe it, even though it was not true. (Please recall the prior discussion of imprinting; therapists have the capacity to imprint, too.) And would it not be possible if the therapist continued to imply (suggest), "Once you have talked about this enough, you will be free of your symptom," the patient would eventually follow the suggestion and be "cured"?

It seems possible, and anyone familiar with the placebo effect in other fields of medicine may not find it difficult to imagine. The fact that it is possible does not mean this is what does happen, but it is a legitimate question and should not be disregarded lightly. After all, the only "proof" supporting the belief that working with Oedipal issues in the hypothetical case effected the cure is the patient's improvement following the use of that technique. That is the same "proof" used to justify the hypnotic technique.

In the actual case, the patient produced data without being led to some foregone conclusion. To label these data as a defense against recognition of the "true" dynamics and to accept data as valid only if they conform to what the therapist's theoretical background says they should be is not consistent with objectivity and basic rules of logical deduction.

I do believe Oedipal and Electra conflicts do exist and may even be universal, at least in our own society, but their occurrence prior to the onset of a symptom does not lead to the logical conclusion that they were the cause of the symptom. Those of us using hypnotic techniques have found, in the great majority of cases, that there was some more specific and mundane traumatic incident or situation which gave rise to the symptoms. This is certainly true in the phobias we work with, just as it was in the case of Little Hans, although in the latter case the historical fact was ignored in favor of theoretical considerations. We have found that, once the trauma is uncovered and the attendant affect recaptured and reduced, then the patient improves. If that sounds familiar, it should, for it is only a slight paraphrasing of what Freud wrote while he was still working with hypnosis.

It is interesting to speculate why those simple procedures appear to work better today than they did for Freud. The techniques are better today, as was mentioned previously, but aside from that, there is another intriguing possibility: Freud's patients did not go back to their real trauma; they went to what Freud presumed their trauma would be. There is no solid evidence to support this conjecture, but let me offer reasons for venturing it.

We know the hypnotized subject will often do or say what he believes the operator expects of him; for instance, Mesmer's subjects, expecting a flow of energy or fluid from Mesmer's hands to their bodies, reported seeing that flow. We do not know why his early patients had "crises," but he became convinced the crises were therapeutic, he encouraged them, patients expected them, and large numbers of patients displayed them. I do not know why the first childhood sexual trauma cases of Freud revealed childhood sexual trauma; perhaps they had actually experienced them. (Success with his earlier cases encouraged him to continue the use of hypnosis for several years.) It is quite conceivable that, once it became known that Freud was expecting to find similar trauma in his hysterical patients, his patients commenced reporting similar trauma, even when they did not exist. The poor therapeutic results that followed further discouraged Freud in his use of hypnosis.

To return to our current methods: Although the next two chapters will deal with techniques for attenuating affect and for helping the patient "work through" his neurosis, I should point out that those techniques are often unnecessary after using ego state therapy. In the first chapter I listed the four important steps I believe to occur in successful insight-oriented therapy: recovery of repressed material, a reexperiencing of the affect associated to that material, attenuation of the affect, and learning how to face new situations unencumbered by the incidents and affects that had been repressed. Using the last case illustration—that of Robert—as an example, perhaps we can see how those four steps were accomplished in one session.

The case of Robert does not demonstrate all the steps as distinctly or dramatically as other cases might; still, they are there and can be recognized. In this case, repressed material and the attendant affect are one and the same. Robert was conscious of the fact that he and his family had moved when he was six, but the terrible pain he had suffered when he left his friends and his pets behind had been repressed. Under hypnosis, the part, Monster, was immediately aware of the pain and reexperienced it, although to a much lesser degree than it had been felt earlier. The affect was attenuated both by the reexperiencing of it and by the simple supplying of new data: Robert is much bigger now, the events happened a long time ago and he no longer has to suffer from them—he is not faced with the same danger of leaving loved ones behind. Learning how to face new situations was accomplished initially by suggesting that intimate relationships could provide both pleasure and protection and by his experiencing this to be true when he tried it out during the week following the session.

Perhaps this sounds too simple to be believable, but a careful, open-minded examination of the steps involved will most likely demonstrate that aside from the use of hypnosis and a more rapid response, nothing occurred that doesn't occur in a traditional therapy. It is true, perhaps, that many therapists would not tell their patients directly that intimate relationships provide pleasure and protection, but they would tell them indirectly by asking, "Do you believe intimacy always involves danger?" or "Can you imagine there might also be benefits to intimate relationships?"

Critics might object to telling the patient such an obvious fact and maintain that the patient's sense of self-accomplishment is diminished by his being told instead of coming to his own conclusions. There may be some truth to the objection, but from experience with many patients, it can now be asserted that the sense of accomplishment arising from ridding oneself of a painful symptom in one week far outweighs the theoretical objections. It should also be noted that Monster came to the conclusion that intimacy was safe after first being told it was and then trying it out for himself.

Removing a Part

Although the basic aim of ego state therapy is to integrate the functioning of the various parts, there was one instance in which I found it necessary to "eliminate" one part that was murderous in its intent toward the patient.

Donna was a severely, suicidally depressed woman in her forties who had made several suicide attempts, had been hospitalized on a number of occasions, had received every antidepressant available, and had received two courses of ECT, all to little avail. Her therapist was retiring and referred her to me.

Donna was an intelligent, articulate woman who had been married to a prosperous and religious businessman who had furthered his business career by inducing her to go to bed with business associates. She left her husband when his own sexual activity became increasingly sadistic toward her. In the divorce proceedings he managed to leave her virtually penniless. She was living with an artist, who seemed to be a kind and gentle man but whose lack of concern about income left them in constant financial straits. Her church, in which her husband was active, excommunicated her for fornication.

When she first came to my office she was not imminently suicidal

but was still in a severe depression and was having recurrent suicidal ideation. The first two sessions were spent gathering her personal history and discussing some of the immediate reality problems
she was facing, including her wish to leave the artist but her fears
of being alone if she did.

During the third session she was introduced to hypnosis, proved
to be an excellent subject, and was taught self-hypnosis as a means
of producing some comfort while we attempted to work on the
underlying problems. Ego state therapy was explained to her and
she expressed her willingness to try it at the next session.

During the fourth session she was put into a hypnotic state, and I
asked to speak with that part which caused her to remain so severely
depressed. "Avenger" came out. Avenger had first appeared when
she was being initiated into her terribly demanding religion, and
this part demanded that she die for violating the tenets of that
religion. All efforts to reason with that part, to bring about a for-
giveness, or at least a less harsh punishment, failed.

Not knowing what else to do, I said to the Avenger, "Since you
are being so unreasonable in demanding the death penalty for a
crime that has hurt no one, I will not let you go back to where you
came from. You must leave her until you're willing to become more
forgiving. When I count backward from three, she will awaken
and you will be gone. Three, two, one, zero, awaken."

Donna let out a shriek, as though something had been pulled
out of her, opened her eyes, stared into the distance for a few moments, and commented, "I feel very different, as though a pain
has gone." She phoned me a few days later to report she couldn't
believe it, but she was no longer depressed. Relieved of her depression, within the next several weeks she left the artist, found a well-
paying job, and several months later met another successful businessman whom she later married. Occasional phone calls over the
next year revealed no return of the depression.

I can offer no good explanation of what occurred here. My pre-
sumption is that the rapport developed via the few sessions of hypnosis enabled her to identify with and introject the less punitive
superego I offered and to use it to replace the murderous superego

she had previously introjected. This is a process which I believe occurs to greater or lesser degrees in most psychotherapies, but rarely so dramatically.

If this technique can so rapidly alter the superego, there could be legitimate concern about the potential for abuse. Again, I do not believe any hypnotic technique will compel a patient to do anything he is unwilling to do, so any alterations in the superego would need to be in those directions the patient was willing to accept. Certainly Donna was more than willing to accept this alteration.

Miscellaneous Thoughts about Ego State Therapy

The concept of there being different parts of the psychic network within us was not new to the Watkins, nor was it new to Federn. Freud, when speaking topographically, referred to the conscious, the unconscious, and the preconscious. When speaking structurally, he referred to the id, ego, and superego.

There was no compelling reason for Freud to call the parts id, ego, and superego. He could have called them Willie, Gladys, and Fred. Admittedly, although a rose by any other name smells just as sweet, a superego named Fred sounds foolish and grates upon our scientific sensibilities. A point could be made, though, that our sensibilities are less important than our patients' improvement. "Superego" as a concept is valuable, but as a name for a punishing part within the patient, it is impersonal and entirely intellectual. If a harsh, punishing part within a patient is named Fred by that patient, the name becomes more personalized and will have some significant emotional meaning to the patient. The therapist may or may not find the meaning if he does look, but emotional associations exist nonetheless. For the patient to have this emotional connection, even at an unconscious level, to the part which has been punishing him is more valuable therapeutically than for him to speak with great sophistication of the punitive superego derived from his obsessive, materialistic, puritanical father. Thus, the names should not be objectionable.

When I think of our great tendency to relish complicated, convoluted theory and highly technical terms, most of which were really neologisms until we accorded them scientific respectability, I am reminded of a humbling passage from Steinbeck's *The Log from the Sea of Cortez.*

> . . . It has seemed sometimes that the little men in scientific work assumed the awe-fullness of a priesthood to hide their deficiencies, as the witch-doctor does with his stilts and high masks, as the priesthoods of all cults have, with secret or unfamiliar languages and symbols. It is usually found that only the little stuffy men object to what is called "popularization," by which they mean writing with a clarity understandable to one not familiar with the tricks and codes of the cult. . . . Can it be that the haters of clarity have nothing to say, have observed nothing, have no clear picture of even their own fields? A dull man seems a dull man no matter what his field, and of course it is the right of the dull scientist to protect himself with feathers and robes, emblems and degrees, as do other dull men who are potentates and grand imperial rulers of lodges of dull men.

The number of parts found within a given patient will be variations of both the intrapsychic conflicts and the therapist's actions. If there be more than three parts, and if those parts do not coincide neatly with the concepts of id, ego, and superego, there should be no cause for dismay. There is no more reason to believe the psyche is composed only of the first three elements found than to believe neurotransmitters are limited to the first few discovered.

I do not know precisely what it means for the therapist to be able to call forth only one part that causes many self-destructive behaviors versus many parts, each of which causes one special self-destructive behavior. My assumption is this: The patient has a number of ego states and each ego state may have had a number of related experiences. The part may have learned at one time that reckless driving brought parental attention; at some later date there was the discovery that the use of cocaine brought forth more parental attention, etc. The patient, complying with the therapist's suggestions, will then produce one unified ego state if requested to do so, or will give names to each of the substates formed with each new but related experience.

The gender of the parts is interesting. As mentioned previously, the gender often seems based on stereotyped concepts of what is male or female. I can offer no further explanation, but I will offer an amusing anecdote. While pondering the whole question of "parts" in a self-hypnotic state, I asked to speak with the female part of myself. "Carol" announced her presence, and I asked her, "Why do I have a female part?" Her response, which seemed to be a gentle mocking of me was, "That's a dumb question. When you were conceived, half of your cells came from your mother; why shouldn't there be a female part?" I asked, "Why, then, did I develop into a male rather than a female?" She replied, "That has all kinds of things to do with chromosomes and hormones, and I don't know. You're the doctor, you should know."

The nature of the work done with ego state therapy raises the specter of the patient developing looser ego boundaries, having problems with dissociation outside of therapy, and becoming relatively disintegrated. In fact, this has not been seen to happen; quite the converse is true. Patients report, "I no longer feel like I'm being pulled in three different directions at the same time," or "I no longer feel like there's a battle raging within myself." The clichéd expression, "I've got to get myself together," vividly describes what needs to be accomplished, and patients indeed feel they have gotten their selves together.

CHAPTER FIVE

Techniques for Attenuating Affect

****

In this chapter we will look at three specific techniques: direct suggestion, implosive desensitization, and silent abreaction. All three of these techniques are relatively mechanical, are not intended for the discovery of new data, and therefore do not offer the excitement of exploration found with the uncovering techniques. As a consequence, they can be relatively dull for the therapist, but the patient, experiencing the affects, finds considerable drama in them. These techniques are not always required, for the uncovering techniques frequently produce sufficient diminution of affect by themselves. There are many cases, however, in which the attenuating techniques have great utility or may even be the primary focus of therapy.

DIRECT SUGGESTION

This is the oldest of all hypnotic techniques, and one of the few

103

available in Freud's time. It is a basic ingredient of all hypnotherapy, as it may be for traditional therapy. ("I wish to speak with the part that . . .," versus, "Tell me what thoughts come to mind." Or "Now that you know where this fear came from, perhaps it won't bother you anymore," versus, "You might feel better if we talked about. . . .")

Direct suggestion is the major component of all hypnotic inductions—for example, "You will become more and more relaxed with every breath," and "As your hand sinks back to the arm of the chair you will find yourself sinking into a state of peace and tranquility." These suggestions seem to work, for the patient looks more relaxed and later reports he felt more relaxed. If these and similar suggestions work with a patient just entering the state of hypnosis, it is to be expected they would work even better with a patient already deeply within a trance state.

Feelings of relaxation are certainly more comfortable than some of the other feelings we experience, so there is more motivation for achieving relaxation. Nonetheless, feelings of a less comfortable nature can also be experienced in response to direct suggestion. Not only can a variety of feelings be experienced, but they can also be diminished or removed, at least temporarily. To whatever extent a feeling may be altered by suggestion in the therapist's office, it may be altered to a greater extent or for longer periods of time by teaching the patient self-hypnosis and instructing him to use autosuggestion for controlling his own responses.

The fact that the patient learns he has the capacity to control himself in this manner can be therapeutic in itself, for he suddenly sees he has the ability to exert some control over his own life and no longer feels as though everything he experiences is the handiwork of some malevolent god. On more than one occasion this has proven to be a major turning point in the patient's therapy.

In looking at the affects which can be attenuated effectively by direct suggestion, it seems that conscious affects arising from consciously recognized sources are the prime targets. If either the affect or its source is unconscious, uncovering techniques should be utilized first.

Case Illustration

Glenda came for help because she felt her whole life was falling apart, everything was going wrong, and she had no control over any of it. She was a poorly educated 28-year-old woman, recently separated from her husband, trying to raise three children on her own. Her husband was still coming around occasionally, breaking down her door or smashing windows; on one occasion he had fired several pistol shots into the ceiling. Her children were in almost constant uproar. She couldn't find a job, largely because she drank herself to sleep each night and arose too late the next day to look for one. She was terribly anxious all the time, to such an extent that she was unable to concentrate on any plan of action.

When hypnosis was mentioned as a possible means of allaying some of her anxiety, she leapt at the chance to use it. A trance state was induced with immediate relaxation becoming evident, and she was taught self-hypnosis as a means of relaxing herself. She was given the direct suggestions that she could now produce relief on her own without the need for doctors or medication, and that being able to control this part of her life would enable her to start regaining control over other portions of her life.

By the second visit beneficial results were apparent. Glenda was feeling much calmer, was sleeping well without alcohol, was no longer anxious all day long, had made definite plans to move to her mother's home in another county as a temporary refuge, and had lined up several possible jobs as a waitress in local but fancy bars. She attributed the change to the realization that if she could control one aspect of her life, she could control other aspects as well.

By the next week she had made her move, had found work, and was enjoying a much happier relationship with her children. For the next three weeks she came into the office primarily to report further progress she had made and to discuss better methods for dealing with her children. By the sixth visit she felt she could handle things on her own again, and we terminated.

Another Case Illustration

Heidi was a well-educated woman in her mid-forties who was referred by an internist because of a simple phobia. She was becoming increasingly frightened of riding the local rapid transport system and would lose her job if she became unable to ride it. A brief history revealed that her symptoms had commenced shortly after a flight from Europe during which bad weather and engine trouble had produced marked anxiety. Anxiolytic agents prescribed by her internist had done little to give her any relief. She had had no prior psychiatric difficulties and appeared basically healthy in all other regards. Financial considerations and the incompatibility of our work schedules made a series of sessions impractical.

Hypnosis was offered as a possible means of helping her overcome her phobia quickly, and although she was initially hesitant about being hypnotized, after a brief discussion of her unwillingness, she agreed to try it. She went into a trance state easily and was taught to do self-hypnosis. She was then rehypnotized and given direct suggestions that she could use self-hypnosis to relax herself before entering the station, that she would feel more comfortable in the stations and on the trains, and that she would reach her destination safely, just as she had landed safely after her flight from Europe. The entire treatment took one standard session.

Telephone follow-up two weeks later revealed she was doing much better. Two months later she was having a mild recurrence of her symptoms, but with one more session to reinforce the previous suggestions and to reinforce her ability to do self-hypnosis, further improvement was obtained, and recent follow-up indicates she is using the transit system comfortably.

Discussion

In the first case illustration the sources of anxiety were undoubtedly evident: multiple situational disturbances which had become overwhelming. In the second case I believed the source of the phobia was also evident—the flight from Europe. Here, though, there will be great disagreement from the traditional therapist. Traditional therapy maintains phobias do not originate from such plebeian origins. Repeated experience has led me to believe they do. More often than not, the source of the phobia is within conscious recollection, although the patient may not have made a conscious connection between the source and the symptom. In long-standing phobias, particularly those which have been present since childhood, the source may have been repressed, but uncovering techniques will usually reveal a very specific incident. To illustrate, I will list a few of the cases that come to mind:

1) Agoraphobia with panic attacks—originated from near asphyxiation from a bolus of food.

2) Agoraphobia with panic attacks—originated from a doctor telling the patient, mistakenly, that he had multiple sclerosis, a disease the patient knew to be fatal.

3) Agoraphobia—originated from a brutal beating sustained when an intruder entered the home at night.

4) Claustrophobia—originated from a rape and beating when the patient stepped out of the shower and was attacked by an intruder.

5) Claustrophobia—originated from the sensation of smothering when the patient, as a three-year-old, had a blanket thrown over her. This was a repressed memory revealed by one of the uncovering techniques. More will be said about this case shortly.

7) Acrophobia—resulted from the mother's frantic screams as the patient, while still an infant, crawled toward an open window. This was another repressed memory revealed by one of the uncovering techniques.

8) A driving phobia—resulted from humiliating taunts when the patient, then a teenager, refused to play "chicken" in his automobile. This case also will be discussed briefly in the next section.

It will be noted, of course, that I claim these incidents were the origins of those phobias but can offer no proof of their being anything more than screens for the real dynamics. That is true, but this much can be said: In none of the cases had the patient made a conscious connection between the incident and the symptom; the connections were made most frequently by ideomotor responding, but in a few instances by other uncovering techniques; after attenuation of the affect associated to the original trauma, the phobia disappeared; follow-up, as long as five years later in one case, three years later in another, and at least several months later in all, revealed no return of the original symptom and no symptom substitution.

IMPLOSIVE DESENSITIZATION

This technique is approximately the reverse of progressive desensitization as used by the behavioral therapists. In progressive desensitization the patient is first trained in relaxation techniques (or hypnotic relaxation may be induced) and is then given a hierarchy of progressively disturbing scenes. If, for instance, the patient were being treated for fear of large gatherings of people, he would be instructed to make a list of all aspects of that situation which might be disturbing to him and then arrange the list in order of increasing disturbance: being with three close friends, being with five or six people, some of whom he didn't know, and so forth, to the point of being at a large banquet and finding himself called upon to make a speech.

First the patient would be relaxed and then instructed to imagine scene number one as vividly as possible and to raise his hand if he began to become anxious. If he could handle the first scene without anxiety, he would then be given the second scene to imagine, and so on, until his hand raised. At that point he would be given instructions for relaxation again, and no further advances in the hierarchy would be made until the next visit. As the patient became able to handle increasingly difficult scenes in his imagination, he would soon become able to translate his mastery of the imagined scene into mastery of real life situations that were similar.

I either laugh or cringe whenever I think of using this technique, not because of any fault with the technique but because of a personal embarrassment during my first year of residency. I had been assigned a patient who had been admitted to the inpatient service following a suicide attempt. Although there were other highly significant problems in her life, she attributed her depression to her fear of having sex with her husband. I was unable to elicit much useful data about her fear and, having recently attended a conference on behavior therapy, decided to try progressive desensitization.

I instructed her to make a list of progressively frightening incidents involving her fear and offered examples: walking down the street and seeing your husband; walking beside him in broad daylight; holding hands as you enter a room with other people, etc.

The following day, the social worker who had just had an interview with the husband reported he was ready to punch me out. He told the social worker I had instructed his wife to make a list of twenty reasons she didn't like to have intercourse with him, and his wife had become upset because she could think of only thirteen. That night they had intercourse, and as soon as they finished her face brightened up and she said, "Now I can think of seventeen."

I would like to believe this is not the only reason I prefer using implosive desensitization; it seems to me the latter is actually more efficient. Instead of starting with a mildly disturbing scene and gradually building up to more disturbing ones, implosive desensitization employs the original affect present at the time of the traumatic incident and has the patient relive it several times until it is markedly diminished. The reader may note a similarity between this technique and the affect bridge. The primary difference is that the affect bridge is used to recover memory of a past traumatic episode, while the desensitization is used to alleviate the affect connected to a trauma which has been remembered.

An age regression technique is used to accomplish this. For instance, the patient is hypnotized and told, "When I count backward from ten, you will be reexperiencing that terrible flight back from Europe. You will be there, seeing it, hearing it, and feeling all the fear you had at the time. Ten, nine. . . ."

The first time the patient reexperiences the original affect, the impact may be quite severe and is easily discernible by the facial and bodily expressions. When this occurs, the experience may be interrupted within the first ten or fifteen seconds by suggesting, "Now the scene is fading away . . . it is gone . . . and you are relaxing again, deeply, comfortably relaxed." If the patient's response is less intense, the event may be permitted to last for thirty seconds, sixty seconds, or longer. I personally allow at least one or two minutes of relaxation between scenes; the more intense the experiencing of the affect, the longer the relaxation permitted before going through it again.

Before having the patient reexperience the affect a second time, I prefer asking the patient if he is willing to do so, explaining to him that this time the affect will probably be less intense and will become even milder with each subsequent episode. This is another example of a question which is partly superfluous, because the patient would not follow the suggestion were he not willing, but the question reassures the patient that the therapist is aware of and concerned about any discomfort the procedure produces. The explanation about an expected reduction of intensity is more than just an explanation; it is also a suggestion for reducing the intensity.

After the patient has been through the scene three or four times and is feeling only slight discomfort with each repetition, a positive aspect of the scene is built into it. As examples of the positive structuring, I will use the case of claustrophobia resulting from the blanket being thrown over the little girl's head and the case of the driving phobia mentioned in the previous section.

Blanket Case

Lucille originally sought help because she and her husband wanted to have children, but she was afraid of getting pregnant. A brief exploration of her fear revealed she had a generalized claustrophobia and knew that when a woman went into labor she was required to ride the elevator to the delivery floor. The fear of the elevator ride was the real fear, not the pregnancy. An uncovering technique restored her memory of feeling terror when she was a little girl of three and her father threw a blanket over her as she was playing on the floor.

Implosive desensitization was used. After repeated relivings of the scene had eliminated almost all emotional response to it, the positive suggestion was made, "This time when you reexperience the sensation of your daddy throwing the blanket over you, you will feel quite differently. You will know he is there to help you if you need help, so you'll be perfectly safe. You'll know he's only playing this silly game because he loves you and believes you'll enjoy the game. This time, then, you'll be able to laugh and giggle because the daddy who loves you is playing a game with you." (The patient laughed and giggled the next time she reexperienced the scene.) The entire treatment required two sessions. Follow-up three years later revealed she had become pregnant, had delivered without incident, and had had no return of her symptoms.

Driving Case

Phillip sought help because he had a phobia about driving an automobile and this seriously interfered with his ability to find a job. Originally, he gave me a story about having survived a fatal accident and having developed a fear of driving after that. The story sounded too pat and too clichéd, so I told him there was something about the story that didn't ring true. He readily admitted it wasn't true, but it had served as a plausible excuse when other people asked him about his fear. He didn't know where the fear had come from.

An uncovering technique was used, and he was brought back to a scene in his teenage years. He and some friends had met one Saturday night, and his friends had challenged him to some dangerous games involving speeding cars down the highway. He refused and was subjected to cruel taunts about his being a coward. His phobia developed soon after that. The incident itself had been available to conscious recall, but he had never made the connection between the incident and the phobia.

Implosive desensitization was used and after he no longer felt more than a slight trace of humiliation, the positive suggestion was given: When he reexperienced the scene the next time, instead of feeling humiliated he would feel proud of himself for having had the intelligence to refuse to play the stupidly dangerous game, and he could be proud of his courage in refusing to play it even though he knew his friends would make fun of him. The entire treatment took two sessions. A week later he reported driving several hours a day just for the fun of driving, and a follow-up five years later revealed he had gotten a job shortly after the end of therapy and had had no trouble since.

SILENT ABREACTION

I first heard this technique described by Donald Schafer. An abreaction, of course, is a reexperiencing of a powerful emotion, and the person reexperiencing it may make a lot of noise. He may cry, scream, shout, etc., whatever is appropriate to the situation. I have heard one therapist describe using four aides to hold the patient down during an abreaction, and the four might be struggling strenuously for over an hour until peace reigned again. Dr. Schafer worked in an office building where the walls were not soundproof, and to prevent his neighbors from hearing crying, screaming, shouting, etc., he developed this technique. In many ways it appears similar to the technique just described, but it seems to give the patient more a sense of having "let the feeling out" than of passively immunizing himself to it. A minor variation of the technique will be described.

The patient is hypnotized and then told to imagine himself in a large, comfortable, secluded room into which no one may enter without his permission. No one else may see or hear what happens within the room, and no one else will ever know, unless the patient chooses to tell them. When the patient imagines himself in the room he is asked to nod his head in affirmation. The patient is then told there is a television set at the other end of the room and is instructed to nod his head when he sees it.

The patient is told the television screen will light up when the therapist counts to three, and then some very special scenes will come onto the screen. The screen will show images of himself expressing his feelings toward whoever was involved. After counting to three, the therapist may elaborate about the flow of feelings: "The anger is rolling out, boiling out, spewing out, like lava from a volcano," etc. This venting of the affect may continue for some predetermined period, or the therapist may instruct the patient to give a signal when he feels the intensity has diminished.

Some patients are unable to visualize themselves on the screen, and others cannot visualize the object of their feelings; they may, however, "feel" what is happening on the screen, and that works out just as well. Some patients visualize the scene as though it were happening in the present, others as if they were expressing the feelings at the time the feelings first arose. Often the emotions are expressed in a most primitive, brutal fashion, with the object of the anger being mutilated horribly. Because these primitive expressions can be frightening and guilt-provoking to some patients, I generally offer a brief preamble, explaining that this can happen but it should be no cause for concern; whatever appears on the screen is only the unconscious manifestations of long-repressed feelings and has nothing to do with the way in which the patient would actually behave. One or several viewings of the scene cause a great release of pent-up affect, with the patient expressing an immediate sense of relief.

Following this procedure, the patient is often able to face new situations with an entirely different feeling state. The emotions which had arisen from his past no longer interfere with his reactions in the present. Not only is he able to behave differently in his outside life, but he also becomes able to reveal more historical data that had been defended against because of the painful affect attendant to those data.

CHAPTER SIX

Relearning Techniques

In traditional psychotherapy there is a working-through process which follows the interpretations of impulses and defenses. A single interpretation will often produce important insights but will rarely completely alter patterns of perceptions, feelings, and activities. Repeatedly, the patient will present similar patterns, manifest, perhaps, in different shapes and colorings, but similar patterns nonetheless. Repeatedly, the therapist will make another interpretation, or lead the patient to making it himself, and over a period of time new insights are gained and new patterns emerge—better patterns, we hope, than the old.

A similar process may occur when hypnotherapy is used. There are, however, hypnotic techniques that seem to reduce the period of working-through, sometimes to a single session. The three of special significance are: direct suggestion, fusion of extremes, and hypnotic imagery.

DIRECT SUGGESTION

When an important insight has been achieved via one of the uncovering techniques, a simple, direct suggestion can easily be incorporated into the session while the patient is still in trance: "Now that you understand the origin of this fear (shame, anger, pain, or whatever is appropriate), you will soon be able to overcome it." This, of course, is rather similar to the nonhypnotic suggestion, "Perhaps you'll feel better if we talk about this some more."

In giving such a suggestion while the patient is hypnotized, it is preferable for the therapist to offer indefinite phrases like "soon," rather than "tomorrow at 12:15." The indefinite phrase gives the patient an opportunity to do the working-through at his own pace, and according to his own interpretation of the phrase. "Soon" will mean a few minutes to some subjects, a few hours to others, or even days or weeks to a small percentage.

Since I attach a suggestion like this to all the uncovering work I do, I cannot be certain if the uncovering produced most of the results or if the suggestion was really beneficial. I do know when I've tried suggestions without the uncovering, the results have usually been poor, as Freud discovered much earlier. If such a simple suggestion attached to the uncovering process is truly useful, one must wonder how it effects its importance? One possibility lies in the fact that the patient has just gone through a significant emotional experience, so the suggestion readily becomes an imprint. The imprint, combined with whatever power a hypnotic suggestion has on its own, may add up to sufficient strength to carry the battle. The traditionalist may interpret the improvement as mere transference cure, and he may be correct. If he is correct, no apology to the patient is required: The unresolved transference will not hamper the patient's life. The unresolved symptom would.

The Case of Paul

Paul is a ten-year-old boy who was referred by another therapist for treatment of an hysterical paralysis of both legs. The patient, who had been paralyzed for two weeks, had had a medical workup which showed no organic origin for his symptoms. He was a pleasant, intelligent, effeminate-looking youngster who did not appear distressed by his illness but who protested convincingly that he wanted to be able to get out of his wheelchair so he could go out and play again.

Ideomotor responses indicated the source of his symptom was a conflict: His brother had been teasing him badly and he wanted to kill his brother. His brother was larger and older than he, and the patient feared the brother would kill him if he tried. (It was my distinct impression he was talking figuratively rather than literally about the killing.) A silent abreaction was used to attenuate the angry affect. Usually, four or five minutes will suffice to diminish the affect sufficiently, but this patient watched the destruction of his brother on the imagined television screen for a full twenty minutes before he was satisfied. Simple suggestions were given: "Now that you are not so angry, there's no need to hurt your brother; you'll find better ways to handle his teasing; you'll be able to use your legs again when you're ready."

Paul was seen again one week later. He reported his paralysis had disappeared about two hours after our first session, and he said he was feeling fine since then. He realized the teasing his brother and classmates gave him was only a game to make him angry, and he learned to ignore it. He also reported an entirely new behavior; now if a classmate pushed him around, instead of passively accepting the push, he would push back, and he found that caused the classmate to stop picking on him. He did not feel that he had any other problems to discuss, so we terminated.

Two weeks later his mother reported continuing good results and canceled further sessions with the prior therapist. Two months later he was still doing well. There has been no further follow-up.

Direct suggestion in the absence of first uncovering a repressed dynamic or a repressed connection to a conscious dynamic is not likely to produce such good results. There are exceptions, however, for at times there are no underlying dynamics or the dynamics no longer possess significant force. Bad habits, like fingernail biting or cigarette smoking, are good examples of this.

Either habit may have started as a conscious or unconscious identification with important persons in the patient's life, but continued identification holds little current appeal. Either habit may have started as an anxiety-relieving measure for external stresses that no longer exist. Either may have started to keep something in the mouth as a protection against letting something (bad words) out of the mouth, but that fear no longer remains. Of course, there are numerous other possibilities, but in examples like those listed, direct suggestion will often provide all the therapy needed.

If the habit is more than just a habit—that is, if there are significant dynamic origins and a persisting neurotic need for the symptom—the suggestions will prove relatively futile. The use of ideomotor responses can rapidly and reliably let the therapist know if he is dealing with something more important than just a bad habit. After the patient has been hypnotized and instructed in the use of ideomotor signals, he may be asked: Do you have any need to keep this symptom? If you gave it up, would that cause any problems at this time in your life? Are you willing to give it up? If he answered "no" to the first two questions and "yes" to the third, direct suggestion would probably be effective and there would be no complications following its use.

It is interesting to speculate if the bad habit concept may be far more important than we customarily believe. It seems possible that some of the "neurotic" symptoms we find are similar to the cigarette smoking in that they were the result of dynamics of great import at one period of the patient's life, but the dynamics have long since faded into obscurity and the behavior patterns persist as nothing more than ingrained habitual responses.

Because direct suggestion appears to be less effective when it is not attached to an uncovering process, it is quite useful to teach the patient self-hypnosis and have him repeat the suggestions to himself a number of times each day. This is not as demanding a task for the patient as it might sound. With a little practice, most patients can learn to enter the hypnotic state, repeat their suggestions, and come out of the hypnotic state in less than sixty seconds. Thus, they can do it before arising from the breakfast table, when sitting down after making a phone call, in the car either before starting the engine or after turning it off, in the bathroom, etc. The benefits accrued from these brief periods seem to accumulate throughout the day, but a few longer sessions, three to five minutes in length, seem to add to the effectiveness.

It is also my impression that the suggestions work more effectively when they are connected to rational reasons for accepting them and when they are given in a permissive manner rather than as direct commands. For instance, instead of "Once you leave this office, you'll start throwing up every time you try to insult a customer!" there would be something like this: "The success of your business is important to you and your family at this time in your life. If you continue being rude to your customers, they won't keep coming back, and your business will suffer. Soon you can learn to be more patient and courteous with them."

Again, a reminder: Chances of success in the hypothetical case above are good if the rude behavior is only a lamentable habit for dealing with people. If there are still current and important dynamic reasons for the rudeness, uncovering work done before the direct suggestions would greatly enhance the possibility for success. The Spiegels (1978) offer many fine examples of using direct suggestion without the uncovering process in their book, *Trance and Treatment*.

FUSION OF EXTREMES

Reaction formations, which cause us to behave in one way because we are afraid of behaving in the opposite way, can be helped quickly and effectively with this technique. The therapist who has anything of the playwright in his blood can exercise his imagination in creating scenarios of many different forms, depending upon the situation the patient presents. My case example clearly demonstrates that the playwriting ability need not be of major caliber.

This technique is probably beneficial to the patient because it permits him to realize more easily than he could with nonhypnotic techniques that it is not necessary to go to one extreme because of his fear of going to the other extreme. Stated simply and briefly, the technique involves having the hypnotized patients imagine two different people responding to the same situation in opposite ways and then seeing those two people merge into one, with the one possessing the better characteristics of each and free of the worst characteristics of each. Almost always the patient can easily identify the fused image as the type of person he wishes to be. A brief case example describes more clearly how the technique is used.

The Case of Sharon

Sharon was a highly intelligent graduate student in Slavic languages who initially sought help because she had found herself unable to complete her doctoral thesis. The therapy, which began before some of the uncovering techniques described in this volume were known to me, ranged over many broad areas, including sexual problems, sibling rivalry, and powerfully ambivalent feelings toward both parents. Her ambivalence toward her father included feelings of rage toward him, and her wish to destroy men was the origin of a reaction formation which caused her to "rescue" men time after time. She was able to get revenge on them, at the unconscious level, by being anorgasmic during intercourse but most efficiently orgasmic with self-stimulation.

One session she came to the office in considerable distress. She was to meet with the chairman of her department the following day to discuss her thesis, and she was dreading the encounter. She saw him as a bullying, arrogant man and was frightened she would break down crying in front of him.

She was put into a hypnotic state and told: In a few moments I am going to describe a scene, and as I describe it, you will experience it as though it were a dream. In a dream you can hear things, feel things, and do things, even though you are sleeping quietly. In the same way you will be able to experience what I am going to describe.

There is a man in an office, seated behind a desk, working at some papers. He hears a knock at the door and yells out angrily, "Come in!" The door opens and a small, frightened woman enters. Trembling, she approaches the desk. He sits there glaring at her, waiting for her to speak.

She opens her mouth, but she can't get any words to come out. He looks at her with contempt and says, "My time is too important to waste on a mute. What do you want?" Again she tries to speak, but can only cry. He comes from behind the desk, grabs her shoulders, and starts shaking her. "Speak out! Don't act like such a disgusting, sniveling little worm!" The scene continues with whatever elaboration the therapist chooses until the poor woman is nothing but a lump of garbage relegated to one corner of the room.

The man goes behind the desk and resumes his work. There is another knock at the door. Disgusted, he yells, "Come in!" This time another woman enters; she is huge and powerful-looking, a real Amazon. He makes a nasty comment to her. She looks at him coldly, walks behind the desk, grabs him by the collar, pulls him from his chair and says, "Don't you ever talk to me like that again, you son-of-a-bitch!" The scene is elaborated until she has reduced him to nothing but a cowering, bleeding mess that she spits upon.

Then the Amazon goes over to the frightened woman in the corner, takes her by the hand, and helps her to her feet. As they stand side by side, a strange thing happens. They begin to fuse into one person. The one person is neither as large as the Amazon nor as small as the first woman. She is neither as cowardly as one nor as brutal and destructive as the other. She has the best characteristics of both: strength, but consideration; courage, but compassion, etc.

The patient was brought out of the hypnotic state and exclaimed, "That was such a strange experience! Before you described the second woman I knew she would look like an Amazon, and when you said the two women would become one, I could see myself, and

I began to feel like that one woman. I believe I can handle the interview now."

The next day Sharon phoned to report that she handled herself well, and there were never any further reported difficulties of the kind with her chairman. The results, however, did not generalize to her relations with other men. Her anger at them, her wish to hurt them, and her reaction formation which caused her to rescue them continued until we had worked it through via other techniques. In retrospect, I can only wonder why I did not try this same technique in a more generalized setting.

Because this patient was so bright and perceptive, I did not add the simple suggestion I would have added for most patients before ending the trance state. Usually, I would have said, "As you think about the one woman who was formed from the two, you will realize you are very much like her. You have the better characteristics of each and do not have to act like the worse side of either. Soon you will begin to feel more and more like the combination and will find it easier and easier to act as she would."

HYPNOTIC IMAGERY

Another method of helping patients learn to do whatever they wish to do, in whatever manner they wish to do it, is to have them imagine doing it correctly while in a hypnotized state. Kroger and Fezler (1976) have written a number of fantasy images which can be used for this and other purposes. The therapist can read the images to the patient directly from the book or can memorize and recite them, but that diminishes the flexibility, does not allow individual variation to suit the particular patient, and deprives the therapist of the opportunity of inventing his own, with whatever elaboration he chooses. This technique is similar to the fusion of extremes but differs in these regards: It is not limited to describing scenes at opposite ends of a spectrum, it can be used to imagine very realistically an actual situation, or it can be used symbolically in describing a desired feeling or behavior. Again, a case presentation will be used for illustration.

The Case of Helen

Helen had been in a state hospital for well over a year, with a diagnosis of schizophrenia. When she first came to the office for treatment, she was doing badly in many regards. She was leaving her young daughter at home each night while she went to bars, drinking excessively. She slept most of the day, providing minimal care to her daughter or to her house. She became involved in a series of harmful relationships and was in constant financial distress, preferring to sell off her meager belongings rather than seek any type of employment.

Slowly, she was able to improve in all those areas to a marked degree and displayed no overt evidence of a psychosis. She retained an agoraphobia with panic attacks. The usual uncovering techniques and attempts at diminution of affect were totally unsuccessful. She was taught self-hypnosis and given images of going outdoors comfortably, with instructions to practice those images several times a day. That, too, proved unsuccessful, and hypnotherapy was discontinued. She moved to another community but returned for follow-up visits every month or two.

On one of those visits she declared her life was going well for her, except for the continued agoraphobia. I suggested we try hypnosis again, and she agreed but commented she didn't like the suggestions about having floating feelings, for that was the feeling she had before a panic attack. She wanted to feel more like she had her feet firmly on the ground and, as she continued talking, told me of hating the many moves she had made in her life, for not only did they deprive her of feeling she had permanent roots, but they also made her feel as though she had left a little bit of herself wherever she had lived.

When asked what kind of scene was most relaxing to her, she replied, "A scene at the beach." I hypnotized her and created an image of a beach: There were heavy, massive, immovable boulders resisting the force of the waves and the wind. The boulders were strong and would stand steadfast for eons. When she came out of the trance she told me she didn't like that image at all. It sounded cold and wet, so she had ignored what I was describing and imagined a tree on the land. She did not want to practice with my image, and the next time I saw her there was no improvement in her symptoms.

On the following visit I described a different scene. There was a tall, sturdy redwood, its roots firmly set in the soil, its trunk growing majestically toward the sky and the sun. It had the strength to withstand the storms, and yet its branches were supple enough to bend with the breezes, always returning to their proper positions. Although the tree remained solidly fixed in place, its seeds could travel on the winds, and wherever a seed landed and took root, a part of the tree remained. Always, though, the tree was where it should be, and always it would continue growing toward the sky and the sun.

She enjoyed that image and readily made obvious associations. On her next visit Helen reported she was going out and doing things with only minimal discomfort, preparing herself first by using self-hypnosis briefly to see the tree and to let herself feel its strength and permanence. There was no further follow-up, for I moved my practice and contact was lost.

CHAPTER SEVEN

Putting It All Together

Recovering repressed memories and the affect associated to those memories, attenuating the affect, and helping the patient learn how to face new situations unencumbreed by the effects of his prior experiences and perceptions are the primary goals of an insight-oriented psychotherapy. The preceding chapters have discussed techniques which should enable the therapist to accomplish those tasks more efficiently than he could with the more traditional techniques.

The techniques themselves are easily learned by anyone with enough flexibility and enough interest to give them a try. There is little likelihood of any damage being done if the hypnotherapist is well trained in any of the various schools of psychotherapy. Such training enables the competent therapist to recognize crises and to deal with them in a familiar manner should they arise. Although a crisis produced by hypnotic techniques is no more likely than one produced by other techniques, the possibility always exists, and it seems only logical that no person should attempt any formal therapy without sufficient formal training. Since this logic does not always carry into actual practice, the patient would be well advised to seek therapy only from a therapist with formal training.

Assuming the hypnotist has had formal training in doing psychotherapy, how does he then apply the techniques described? Flexibly! There are no hard and fast rules to govern the selection of techniques nor the sequence of techniques; only general guidelines can be offered. The first is to remember that hypnosis is no magic; like other forms of therapy, it does not always work, and even when it does, it can often be supplemented by other modalities. The use of traditional methods of therapy and the use of medications may be indicated along with the use of hypnosis, and the therapist should employ whatever seems most appropriate at the time.

Selection of Patients

Numerous studies have failed to indicate that any of the traditional personality types are better hypnotic subjects than the others, although there is still the widespread misconception that the obsessive patient is always difficult to hypnotize and the hysterical patient is always easy. Spiegel and Spiegel (1978), after quoting many studies on personality types and hypnotizability, have described three new personality types—Apollonian, Odyssean, and Dionesian—who, in that order, are said to be progressively more easily hypnotized, but the Apollonian seems remarkably like the obsessive personality and the Dionesian like the hysterical personality. With approximately 95 percent of patients being hypnotizable, it doesn't seem to matter much what personality type they are.

Generally, the patient's diagnosis seems much less important than the problem he presents, but there are a few exceptions. The patient suffering from an organic brain disease, including acute intoxication from alcohol, marijuana, or other drugs, is usually a poor subject for hypnotherapy. Patients stoned on marijuana are easily hypno-tized, but the results are unimpressive. Poor concentration, recent memory deficits, and perhaps other impairments as well make it difficult to work with the other causes of organic brain disease.

The schizophrenic patient and the manic patient are poorly suited for hypnotherapy during times of great distractibility; how-ever, during periods of quiescence, they can be hypnotized and can benefit from therapy. I do not expect either could be cured of his underlying illness by means of hypnotic interventions, but these patients are not immune from the less severe problems that beset all of us, and they can receive help in those areas.

The depressed patient with severe psychomotor retardation has proven difficult to hypnotize, but once the psychomotor retardation is relieved, he can be an excellent subject in whom uncovering tech-niques can be highly useful. This patient, like the schizophrenic and manic patients, is a good example of those for whom medications are an important supplementary treatment modality.

The patient who presents primarily with an external, reality-based problem that is correctible has a 95 percent chance of being a good hypnotic subject, but the probabilities are good that nonhypnotic techniques will be equally or more effective in helping him find solutions.

These are the few major exceptions to patients who are most likely to benefit from hypnotherapy. The next question becomes: What techniques should be used for which problems?

Cases Not Requiring Uncovering Techniques

Many patients seek therapy for problems that do not have an important, repressed, underlying dynamic. For these patients, atten-uation of affect, relearning techniques, or simple direct suggestion will be the techniques of choice. Because the therapist may not al-ways know if there are important underlying dynamics or not, be-fore he attempts removing a symptom he should consider at least a brief exploration via ideomotor responding. This was mentioned previously, but to reiterate: The patient is asked, "Does this symptom serve some useful purpose for you? If it were removed, would that cause you any further trouble? Are there any reasons you should not give up this symptom at this time?" If the ideomotor responses are all "no," symptom removal may proceed.

Removal of Bad Habits

The most frequent example is cigarette smoking. Fingernail biting, hair twisting, etc., are other common habits, but rarely have I seen a patient who wished to go to the trouble and expense of relieving himself of this relatively minor problem. I will focus on the smoking habit, and the reader can easily extend the principles to other situations.

The basic principles are: Build an aversion to the undesired behavior, build rewards for desired behavior, alleviate the discomforts of withdrawal, and give direct suggestions that the patient can stop smoking. One other principle I have adopted is to inform the patient I will see him only once, unless he has had at least a three-month "cure" and then slips back. In that case I will see him for one-half session to reinforce what was achieved. Since going from a four- to six-session treatment plan to this one-session treatment plan, results have leapt from about 15 percent success to approximately 60 percent, due, I believe, to the demand for greater motivation on the patient's part.

Some therapists in creating aversion to the undesired behavior produce truly repulsive images for the patient to endure. I do not believe in that; I feel it is unnecessary, constitutes an affront to the patient's dignity, and falls into the realm of suggestions the patient is reluctant to accept. The aversions I use come entirely from the patient's own reasons for wanting to stop smoking. A typical session would include these specific steps:

1) Obtain a brief history of the habit.
2) Obtain *all* the reasons for wishing to stop.
3) Hypnotize the patient once or twice and teach him self-hypnosis.
4) Rehypnotize him and give him the following suggestions:

A. Each time you are tempted to have a cigarette, you will immediately think of all the disgusting things the cigarette means to you (enumerate them). The disgust will greatly diminish your desire to smoke one.

B. Each time you refuse to yield to that temptation, you will be rewarded with a feeling of pleasure and pride that you had the intelligence and strength to stop this disgusting habit.

C. The longer you go without smoking, the more rewards you will accumulate: You will feel healthier, you will have more vitality and stamina, you may find that you think more clearly and have a greater sexual drive. Because your nostrils are not contaminated with smoke, pleasant aromas might be more distinct. Because your tastebuds are not coated with tars and nicotine, food might taste better, but *this will not cause you to overeat!* Because food tastes better, you will get more enjoyment from a smaller amount, and therefore you will not gain weight.

D. When you see others smoking, this will no longer be a temptation to you but will give you a silent pride that you were able to stop a disgusting habit that they have not been able to stop.

E. If you have withdrawal symptoms they will be relatively mild and brief, and you will be able to get through them easily.

F. You can use the self-hypnosis to relax yourself whenever you wish, and you can use it to reinforce any or all of these suggestions.

G. You can stop smoking as of now. You can stop smoking as of now. You can stop smoking as of now!

Engendering Good Habits

There are two basic techniques to use for this purpose: Direct suggestion and visual imagery. With either, the patient would be taught to do self-hypnosis in order to reinforce what was done in the therapist's office. If, for instance, the patient wished to establish better study habits, direct suggestions could include:

1) It is very important for your career and your future happiness that you do well in school.

2) To do well in school, it is important that your study habits improve, and soon they will.

3) When you are ready to study, you will put yourself into a state of self-hypnosis briefly, and when you bring yourself out of it you will find you have greater concentration for one or two hours.

4) This improved concentration will permit you to understand the material more readily and remember it more clearly, so that later you will be able to recall it more easily.

5) You may repeat this process whenever you wish.

For habits that require less mental ability the therapist might have the patient visualize himself behaving in the manner he desires. The scene the therapist describes should be as realistic as possible, with suggestions that the patient not only see himself doing the desired acts but feel himself doing them as well.

Reducing Affect from Known Sources

Problems of this sort fall into two general categories: unpleasant affects engendered by an ongoing situation (i.e., a high-pressure job) and unpleasant affects remaining from some past trauma (i.e., a recent death in the family). In either of those two cases, not only is the source of the affect known, but it is also easily recognized as a rational feeling about a specific situation. The therapist should make no attempt to have the patient deny the affect or to "forget" it; all efforts should only be attempts to help the patient cope with the feelings in a better manner.

For those cases in which there is an ongoing disturbing situation, the patient is taught self-hypnosis and given simple suggestions such as: "When you enter your self-hypnotic state, this feeling of relaxation will return to you and remain with you for a long time afterward. This will enable you to face the situation with greater calmness and comfort." For those cases in which the affect arose from one specific trauma, the silent abreaction is used to diminish the affect and thereby hasten the working-through of the grief, jealousy, anger, etc.

Relieving Insomnia

Here it is particularly important to check via ideomotor responding to see if there is an underlying reason for the symptom. Many cases, however, seem to have none and are therefore easily treated with a combination of visual imagery and direct suggestion. The therapist teaches the patient how to do self-hypnosis and then, while the patient is hypnotized, describes as vividly as possible the patient becoming sleepy at night, making his usual preparations for bed, climbing into bed, feeling the comfort of the sheets and blankets, adjusting his head on the pillow, closing his eyes, and falling into a deep, safe sleep from which he will awaken in the morning feeling rested and well. The simple suggestions are added that he will use the self-hypnosis to repeat this scene for himself, and soon he will be sleeping the way he imagines it in that scene. Good results can frequently be obtained in one or two sessions.

These are the primary cases for which I believe uncovering techniques are unnecessary. Many authors have reported good results using only direct suggestion or visual imagery with a host of other problems. My own experience has been that my own results are greatly improved when the patient and I first discover the origin of the symptom.

SELECTION OF UNCOVERING TECHNIQUES

Although I believe it probable that any of the three uncovering techniques could be used interchangeably, often patients clearly suggest one might be better than another. The patient who spontaneously states, "Part of me wants to do this, but another part wants to do that," is a prime candidate for ego state therapy. Somewhat less obvious variations would be: "Sometimes I . . ., but other times I . . .," or, "I believe . . ., but on the other hand, I also believe. . . ."

Patients with somatic complaints of psychological origin seem to do better with ideomotor responses, which seems reasonable, since they are already using their bodies to express an internal conflict.

Ideomotor responses also seem to work better for patients who are relatively concrete and who have limited imaginations. To me, the ideomotor responses are usually more time-consuming and less interesting than the other techniques, but their efficacy in these patients enables me to override this objection. If an affect of unrecognizable origin is the prime symptom, the affect bridge would be the primary choice.

These generalized observations are merely rough guidelines and, as demonstrated in some of the case examples, a patient may not respond to the first method tried, so another is tried in its place. At times one technique is used for one problem the patient presents and another technique for a different problem in the same patient. At times either the ideomotor responses or the ego state therapy may lead to an affect that cannot be understood, so the affect bridge is used in addition to the other techniques. Flexibility is essential.

SELECTION OF AFFECT ATTENUATION TECHNIQUES

Once the uncovering work has been done, it is easy and natural to add the direct suggestion, "Now that you know where this came from, you will soon have better control over . . .," or "You will soon feel differently about . . .," or whatever suggestion would be appropriate to the situation. Often this will be all that is needed to help the patient undergo marked changes. If not, either the silent abreaction or the implosive desensitization can be used. Although they, too, can be used interchangeably, I have developed a preference for using the implosive desensitization for fear or disgust and the silent abreaction for most of the other negative affects, primarily anger and grief. Simple suggestion is easily added to either of those: "Now that you have reexperienced (seen yourself expressing) this feeling you have bottled up for so long, you will feel free of it at last."

Although it may take two or three sessions to accomplish this diminution of affect, one session is all that is required for the majority of patients. If two or three sessions are needed, I tend to feel a little discouraged, until I remember how long it took with more conventional means.

SELECTION OF RELEARNING TECHNIQUES

As mentioned in the preceding chapter, the fusion of extremes seems ideally suited for the patient with a strong reaction formation. For other situations I prefer other hypnotic imagery, repeated by the patient during his sessions of self-hypnosis. This allows the patient to visualize doing whatever he wishes to do in the manner in which he wishes to do it, and he soon becomes able to translate those images into real life situations.

Patients and nonpatients have all had similar experiences without the use of hypnosis. The most striking one for me involves learning to ski. My instructor would tell me repeatedly what I should be doing, and although my head understood perfectly, my body would not respond properly. It was almost as though my head were saying, "Look, dummy, all you need to do is . . .," and my was body responding, "Go to hell! I'm the one that takes the lumps."

During the several weeks that passed before I was on the slopes again, I would often daydream of skiing the way the instructor told me. Although I was in no formal hypnotic state, in my daydreams I could see the slopes, feel myself shifting weight properly, and experience the skis carving the snow the way they should. The first run of my next trip would inevitably be better than any of the runs on the previous trip, and the improvement was maintained. It was as if genuine practice had occurred, but all in my own head. This type of experience is hardly unique to me, and a major portion of the book, *The Inner Game of Tennis* (Gallway, 1974), is devoted to emphasizing the ability of a student to learn by visualizing himself making strokes the way his instructor did.

This raises an important question: Is hypnosis a necessary part of any of this? Probably not. I work on the assumption that anything done with hypnosis could also be done without it, so it is not necessary; it is only remarkably more efficient. Then, too, the fact that it is more efficient may make it necessary, at least in some cases. There are those patients who have neither the emotional nor financial resources to tolerate prolonged therapy, and they could not benefit from therapy at all unless it were efficient; for them, hypnosis may be necessary.

TERMINATION

Most nonpsychotic patients will accomplish what they wish to accomplish in a maximum of eight to twelve visits, many in two or three. I firmly believe in terminating at that point. It is certainly true there will be other conflicts that have been untouched, but if the patient is feeling no distress from them, the therapist should feel no distress from them either. If he does, perhaps he should see another therapist to treat him for his distress and not subject the patient to further visits to relieve his own discomfort.

The patient's unresolved conflicts will follow one of three different patterns: 1) The work already done on the recognized problem areas will have a ripple effect and lead to a spontaneous resolution. 2) The unresolved conflicts will remain unresolved but will continue to cause no problems. 3) They will cause distress at some later date and can be treated then much more efficiently, if the patient elects to return to therapy.

Many patients do elect to return to therapy to work on problems that surfaced after the first termination. Neither they nor I view a return as a failure; realistically, it is an incomplete success. This is no mere game with semantics, for it was their success at resolving earlier conflicts which permitted them to function at higher levels. At those higher levels they ran into problems they would not have encountered before. They have experienced the pleasure of freeing themselves from old problems; they have enjoyed months or years of functioning on their own without therapy; and they return with a strong sense of confidence that they can resolve the new issues successfully.

Before terminating with a patient, I point out to him that new problems may appear later in his life, and he is welcome to return if he wishes to do so. I often use one of two analogies:

If he had fallen from a tree and broken a leg, he would stop treatment once the leg had healed. If later a car struck him on that leg and broke it again, that would not indicate treatment had failed, only that life had dealt him another severe blow and treatment for the new injury was indicated. Or, if he had a car he couldn't drive because the carburetor was defective, and after he had the carburetor repaired the transmission went out, that would not mean the carburetor repair was faulty. It would mean there was an underlying problem in the transmission which would not have caused him trouble, except for his success in being able to drive again.

Before terminating with a patient, I try to stress the fact that the patient was the one who made the changes occur. Hypnosis was merely a skill he learned in order to help himself understand better the origin of his problems and find a solution to them. It was a skill, like reading, which once learned can continue to be useful in a number of ways throughout his life.

I do this to divest the patient of any misconceptions about his improvement being the work of magic. I believe it is an unnecessary precaution. Patients really know they were the ones who made the changes occur, and hypnosis, though helpful, is a long way from being magical.

Because therapy is usually so brief and so active, there is less opportunity for strong transference feelings to develop and to become a problem in termination. At least it is true that transference feelings do not become a problem. I am less certain about the strength of their development. There are those who say hypnosis itself is the result of strong transference feelings in which the patient assumes the role of a child responding to the commands of an all-powerful parent. Since the subject will not following suggestions he does not wish to follow, I find such a theory degrading to the patient and inaccurately enhancing to the therapist.

CHAPTER EIGHT

❖❖

Conclusion

❖❖

✤✤✤

There is a great and growing dissatisfaction with the traditional modes of insight-oriented therapy. Multiple new therapies have arisen in answer to that dissatisfaction. Some of the newer therapies are based on theories foreign to the Freudian viewpoint: One can scream his way into health, be massaged into health, or be reconditioned into health. Some of the newer therapies are based upon theories more closely akin to Freudian formulations, but the techniques are more active: time-limited therapies that focus on separation issues, short-term therapy that focuses on self-punishment as the primary origin of neurotic symptoms, or "relentless" therapy in which the patient is vigorously challenged as he attempts to employ his customary defenses. There are, of course, numerous other examples, and there should be little doubt that still others will arise in the future.

What I have attempted is to present a systematic approach for utilizing a variety of hypnotic techniques to facilitate therapeutic change. It is my observation that the approach has at least three advantages:

1) It produces change with relative efficiency by promoting the same processes which occur in a more traditional type of therapy.

2) It is far less traumatic to the patient, for there are no prolonged, agonized periods of silence, no shameful confessions to be made, no "accusations" to endure, and no tormenting transferences to be resolved.

3) It is more gratifying to the therapist, for it enables him to be a more active participant during each session and brings him the rewards of a successful termination much more quickly.

In the early portions of this book I mentioned that we often must rely upon personal anecdote rather than acceptable statistics to determine the worth of any system of therapy. Realizing this is not compatible with a scientific approach to decision-making, I regret the lack of statistics to validate my observations, but I am a practitioner, not a researcher. The observations, however, are truly reported and deserve consideration by any therapist who ventures to believe that traditional theory is not sacrosanct, and that traditional psychotherapeutic techniques may not represent the ultimate apogee of the art. He and his patients may be richly rewarded by such consideration.

BIBLIOGRAPHY

✠✠

BANDLER, R., and GRINDER, J. (1973), *Patterns of the Hypnotic Techniques of Milton H. Erickson, M.D.*, Vol. 1. Cupertino, California: Meta Publications.

BERNE, E. (1964), *Games People Play*. New York: Grove Press.

BERNHEIM, H. (1884), *Hypnosis and Suggestion in Psychotherapy*. New York: Jason Aronson, 1973.

BLYTHE, P. (1972). *Hypnotism, Its Power and Practice*. New York: Macmillan Publishing Company, Inc.

BRENMAN, M., and GILL, M. (1971), *Hypnotherapy*. New York: International Universities Press.

BREUER, J., and FREUD, S. (1893), On the Physical Mechanism of Hysterical Phenomena: Preliminary Communication, *Standard Edition*, 2:3-17. London: Hogarth Press, 1955.

BURANELLI, V. (1975), *The Wizard from Vienna*. New York: Coward, McCann and Geoghegan, Inc.

DEWALD, P. (1972), *The Psychoanalytic Process: A Case Illustration*. New York: Basic Books, Inc.

ELMAN, D. (1964), *Findings in Hypnosis*. Clifton, New Jersey: Dave Elman.

ERICKSON, M., ROSSI, E., and ROSSI, S. (1976), *Hypnotic Realities*. New York: Irvington Publishers, Inc.

ESTABROOKS, G. (1957), *Hypnotism*. New York: E. P. Dutton & Company, Inc.

145

FEDERN, P. (1952), *Ego Psychology and the Psychoses.* Edited by E. Weiss. New York: Basic Books.

FRANKEL, F. (1976), *Hypnosis.* New York: Plenum Medical Book Co.

FREUD, S. (1891), Hypnosis. *Standard Edition,* 1:103-114. London: Hogarth Press, 1955.

———— (1909), Analysis of a Phobia in a Five-Year-Old Boy. *Standard Edition,* 10:5-147. London: Hogarth Press, 1955.

———— (1910), Five Lectures on Psychoanalysis. *Standard Edition,* 11:9-55. London: Hogarth Press, 1957.

———— ((1925), An Autobiographical Study. *Standard Edition,* 20:1-74. London: Hogarth Press.

———— (1937), Analysis Terminable and Interminable. *Standard Edition,* 23:216-53. London: Hogarth Press, 1964.

GALLWAY, W. (1974), *The Inner Game of Tennis.* New York: Random House.

GREENSON, R. (1967), *The Technique and Practice of Psychoanalysis,* Vol. I. New York: International Universities Press, Inc.

HILGARD, E. (1968), *The Experience of Hypnosis.* New York: Harcourt, Brace, Jovanovich.

————, and HILGARD, J. (1975), *Hypnosis in the Relief of Pain.* Los Altos, California: Wm. Kaufman, Inc.

KROGER, W. (1977), *Clinical and Experimental Hypnosis.* Philadelphia: J. B. Lippincott Co.

————, and FEZLER, W. (1976), *Hypnosis and Behavior Modification.* Philadelphia: J. B. Lippincott Co.

LeCRON, L. (1970), *Self-Hypnotism.* New York: Signet.

———— (1971), *The Complete Guide to Hypnosis.* New York: Barnes and Noble Books.

LEWIN, K. (1970), *Brief Encounters.* St. Louis: Warren H. Green, Inc.

LOFTUS, E., and LOFTUS, G. (1980), On the Permanence of Stored Information in the Human Brain. *American Psychologist,* 35:5, 409/20.

MALAN, D. H. (1980), *Psychotherapy and Social Science Review,* 14:12, 4-7.

MARCUSE, F. (1959), *Hypnosis: Fact and Fiction.* Baltimore: Pelican Books.

MARMOR, J. (1980), Recent Trends in Psychotherapy. *American Journal of Psychiatry,* 137:4, 409-16.

MEARES, A. (1960), *A System of Medical Hypnosis.* Philadelphia: W. B. Saunders Co.

SCHNECK, J. (1954), Countertransference in Freud's Rejection of Hypnosis. *American Journal of Psychiatry,* 110:928-931.

SPIEGEL, H., and SPIEGEL, D. (1978), *Trance and Treatment: Clinical Uses of Hypnosis.* New York: Basic Books.

STEINBECK, J. (1951), *The Log from the Sea of Cortez.* London: Pan Books, Ltd.

WATKINS, J. (1971), The Affect Bridge: A Hypnoanalytic Technique. *International Journal of Clinical and Experimental Hypnosis,* 19:1, 21-27.

————, and WATKINS, H. (1979), The Theory and Practice of Ego State Therapy, in *Short-term Approaches to Psychotherapy,* H. Grayson, Editor. New York: National Institute for the Psychotherapies and Human Sciences Press.

WOLBERG, L. (1965), *Short-term Psychotherapy.* New York: Grune and Stratton.

WOLPE, J., and RACHMAN, S. (1960), Psychoanalytic Evidence: A Critique Based on Freud's Case of Little Hans. *Journal of Nervous and Mental Disease,* 130:99.

INDEX

�֎✤✤

147